The 5:2 Diet

Meals for One
Cookbook

by Liz Armond

Published in UK by:
Liz Armond
© Copyright 2015 – Liz Armond

ISBN-13: 978-1511977784
ISBN-10: 1511977787

Table of Contents

Introduction

Losing weight can be difficult, and knowing which diet to follow can be even harder. This book will help you use the 5:2 Fast Diet or 2 Day Diet to help you easily achieve your weight loss goals.

Although it is quickly becoming one of the most popular diets to lose and maintain your weight loss there are only a few recipe books on the market today that contain single portion meals that are easy to make and don't use hard to get or expensive ingredients. This cookbook also includes enough varied and interesting breakfast recipes for those that need them on your fasting days.

I have lost a significant amount of weight with this diet and wanted more recipes that fitted in with my busy lifestyle and budget but were still delicious to eat. The recipes here are low calorie and healthy, but they make use of many of the basics in your kitchen cupboards.

This cookbook is also designed to complement my series of 5:2 recipe cookbooks. I have adapted many of my recipes to meet the growing demand for single dieters who don't have the time or patience to scale down standard size recipes. Where the recipe calls for only a percentage of a packet or can, just store excess amounts in fridge, freezer or airtight containers until needed again. Just don't forget to label them or you will end up with lots of pots of unknown foods.

One other thing, I enjoy being creative with my food, and I urge you to do the same. For example, try adding a little more spice or different fruits and vegetables or a different stock. I have included a calorie counter to help you recalculate your changed recipes so you can stay within your calorie limit.

I hope you enjoy the recipes in this book and experience the benefit of having food that is quick and easy to prepare as you watch your excess weight drop away.

Many of the recipes included here can be adapted for non-dieters in your family if you are cooking larger portions. Just add potatoes or pasta or even crusty bread for them.

The recipes are listed alphabetically with the calorie count alongside. This is so you can calculate the number of calories you have remaining, and jump to the recipe you fancy with the relevant count. This should inspire you to stay creative and still have the ability to switch your meals without going over your daily allowance.

Above all else, enjoy your food and the process of cooking it. You are only dieting for two days a week, so it is not necessary to stress yourself about it. You are reducing your calorie intake from 2000/2500 calories a day to 500/600 calories a day, so you **WILL** lose weight.

About the 5:2 Fast Diet

What do you know about the **5:2 Fast Diet**? Although this diet, which is based on intermittent fasting, has not been around as long as some other popular diets, it has proven itself by consistently achieving fantastic results in a very short time. If done properly it will help you lose weight really fast and reach your target weight loss easily.

As you might have guessed, the **5:2 Fast Diet** works exactly as the name suggests. During a 7-day period, you will eat normally for 5 days and then for 2 days you will restrict yourself to about a quarter of your normal daily calorie intake. This approach to dieting has proven to help you avoid getting bored with diet foods or long diets. The way it works it to allow you to eat a diet that is somewhat "normal" for a certain period and then you semi-fast for the other period - hence the name, intermittent fasting.

The **5:2 Fast Diet** has consistently come out on top as the diet with no nonsense eating habits and has the most health benefits over longer term diets. **Intermittent fasting** has been proven to fight the onset of diabetes in pre-diabetic people. Research has shown that glucose levels are lowered in people that semi-fast and in those that only consume water for short periods of time.

Of course, this strategy of intermittent fasting does not mean you can eat all of the super high fatty and calorie enriched foods you want on your 'normal' days, especially if you want to get and stay healthy to live longer. But believe me, this diet will change the way you think about food and will even change your eating habits.

Eating your allotted number of calories on your 5 days of 'normal' eating should still be done with healthy and nourishing foods. There is no diet that helps a person look and feel great by consuming 2000/2500 calories of chocolate cake, double cheese pizza, and sugary carbonated drinks. You should try to eat well-balanced meals that should include whole grains, fresh (organic if possible) vegetables and fruits, and lean proteins.

However, with the **5:2 Fast Diet**, you will not just feel like your old self again, results have shown that you will feel much better and healthier than you have in a long time.

It doesn't matter which days you choose to feed or fast but it is recommended that the fasting days are not done together. Depending on the speed you wish to lose the weight you could adjust the ratio of fasting to feeding days.

For example you could try a 6:1 or 5:2 or 4:3 and so on. When you have reached your ideal weight perhaps then is the time to only fast for one day a week to maintain your target weight, but for now let's assume you have a goal to reach, so we will a look at the normal 5:2 diet in more depth.

On fasting days you can elect to consume all of your calories in one go, or more usual to spread them throughout the day. Breakfast can either be a really low calorie count which means you can probably have a light lunch as well or you can skip it altogether. I found skipping breakfast worked better for me as it didn't kick start my juices first thing and I had no problem lasting until midday lunch. I quite often forgot all about food and went to 1 or 2 o'clock before I realised I was getting hungry. I don't think I could eat breakfast and then have nothing until my evening meal.

There is varying opinion on whether filling up at breakfast or snacking throughout the day is more effective for weight loss. You will find your own preferred method, I tried both and found that splitting my calories between lunch and dinner worked better for me but then I can manage to skip breakfast but you may not be able to.

Drink water, tea or coffee to fill your empty stomach but no sugar and watch your milk intake or you will be eating into your calories. But please don't worry about going over the 500 calories by a little bit because when you do follow this eating plan you will be amazed at how you start to look at everything you eat on your 'normal' days and will in fact eat less anyway.

You could try fizzy water or diet soda and some people have suggested chewing sugar free gum although I found that made me hungry.

On your five normal days you can eat whatever you like within reason. This is not carte blanch to load your system with unhealthy junk food. What you will find is that you are looking at packaging much more than you used to. You will be shocked at the amount of calories in one chocolate biscuit, I know I was. If you think about the calories in that one biscuit and then think of the percentage that biscuit is of your 500 or 600 calorie allowance on your fasting days you quickly come to appreciate why that weight gain crept up on you in the first place.

Remember if the hunger pangs become too much, do something active like going for a walk. You can drink as much water as you like and this will fill you up too. Try a little honey or lemon juice in a glass of warm water, you will soon feel full until your meal is due. If you are doing this with your partner, don't forget to factor in an additional 100 calories if you or your partner is male.

If you are worried about the long term effects on your body, contrary to what some people think, fasting can be a healthy way to lose weight. It can reduce levels of IGF-1 (insulin-like growth factor 1, which can lead to accelerated aging). It can also 'switch' on DNA repair genes as well as reducing blood pressure and lowering cholesterol and glucose levels.

A word of warning, it is not recommended for pregnant women or diabetics on medication. In fact anyone who has health problems or has an existing medical condition is strongly advised to consult their GP first. This is not to say you can't follow this diet, it is just so it can be done under medical advice or supervision.

Finally, keep going by thinking to yourself that this is only for 2 days a week, you are not on a full blown 7 days a week diet for weeks on end or in some cases what seems forever.

Well that's all there is to it, well almost.

Finally, as previously mentioned, if you are interested in other methods of fasting, I do cover this in my book on losing weight through fasting called, **_Fasting Your Way to Health._**

Diet the Healthy Way

So, how do you diet healthily?

Be accountable. Whatever the consequences are, you need to be accountable for your actions and diet for the right reasons. Likewise, be sensitive to the response or reaction of family and friends who you confide in about your plans to reduce your food intake for 2 days a week. It is likely that they might have seen something detrimental in the press or on television about the dangers of not eating normally and will only be showing concern for you and your wellbeing.

Prepare in advance. When you have come to the decision to start any type of diet, do not act on the spur of the moment, it will work much better if you have done your preparation beforehand. Make sure you know what appointments or events are likely to happen before, during and after your fasting day. You don't want to plan one of your fasting days only to find you had forgotten you were having lunch with your best friend or had booked a game of golf. If you don't skimp on the preparation time, your fasting day will most likely go more smoothly and be much more enjoyable and effective.

Understand the effects on your body. If you have managed to read some facts and figures on fasting you will know that your body goes through several distinct phases when you begin to fast, even if it is for just one day. It is possible that during the first few hours, you will feel a little weak, especially if you have decided to go without breakfast. You shouldn't be too alarmed by this as it is natural as your body begins to eliminate the toxins in your system.

Break the fast properly. With the 5:2 fast, you won't have many serious side effects but it doesn't hurt to be prepared. Try not to have a great big fry up the next day as a form of reward. Have porridge or your usual cereal so that you don't waste the previous day of healthy eating.

Who Should NOT Fast?

The 5:2 fast will have very little adverse effect on many of the following groups, but use your common sense

1. Infants and children. There is really no good reason for infants and children to fast. Due to their lack of maturity, they would likely not really understand the spiritual purpose of fasting, and their growing bodies need to take in ample nutrients regularly.

2. Pregnant or nursing women. Most fasts, including the 5:2 should be avoided by women who are pregnant or nursing unless cleared by a Doctor. The baby requires so many nutrients for normal development and is dependent on the mother's proper nutrition to receive those nutrients. You are forcing the unborn baby to fast and can be potentially dangerous to both mother and child.

3. People with Cancer - Do not fast unless you are fasting in an attempt to help yourself heal in which case this should be under direct medical advice. The 5:2 is probably not severe enough for this purpose. Cancer is usually indicative of, amongst other things, an immune system that is not in good shape.

4. People with other health concerns. The 5:2 Fast Diet is a good way to regulate food intake on overweight or obese sufferers and juice fasts may be another option. However check with your Doctor first as he may wish to supervise your weight loss.

5. The Elderly - There is no need for the elderly to fast as their body may not be able to manage such a task but it may not hurt them to lose a little weight for mobility reasons. Again use your common sense and perhaps only try 1 day intermittent fasting to start.

And if anyone still has any concerns or questions, they should always ask their doctor. Remember, fasting is supposed to help bring out the best of health for us.

Useful Cooking Terms

The recipes in this book are all tried and tested and are for single portions. Where you have to open larger cans or packets for the required amount of ingredients you can either store them in small containers in the fridge or even freeze them for future fasting meals.

However, although this book is single portions I do recommend that you cook as big a batch as possible, especially if the recipe is marked as suitable for freezing. That way you always have a quick meal in the freezer or fridge at a time when it is probably your busiest but also your hungriest. If you have something planned and prepared you will be less likely to snack.

The ingredients in this book are given in the standard UK & US measurements and the metric equivalent. You should choose one or the other, but try not to mix.

Recipes use many different abbreviations. Here are the ones used in this book.

Standard UK / US

tsp = teaspoon
tbsp = tablespoon
oz/s = ounce/ s
lb/s = pound/s
fl. oz. = fluid ounce

Metric

ml = millilitres
ltr = litre / liter
g = grams

Teaspoons and tablespoons are level measure.

1 tsp = 5ml
1tbsp = 15ml

Liquid volume conversions

⅛ tsp = 0.5 ml
¼ tsp = 1 ml
½ tsp = 2 ml
1 tsp = 5 ml
½ tbsp = 7 ml
1 tbsp = 3 tsp = 15 ml
2 tbsp = 1 fl oz = 30 ml
4 tablespoons = 60 ml = ¼ cup
90 ml = ⅓ cup
4 fl oz = 125 ml = ½ cup
160 ml = ⅔ cup
6 fl oz = 180 ml = ¾ cup

16 tbsp = 8 fl oz = 250 ml = 1 cup

1 pint = 500 ml = 2 cups

1 litre/liter = 1 quart = 4 cups

Weight Conversions

½ oz = 15g

1 oz = 30g

2 oz = 60g

3 oz = 85g

¼ pound = 4 oz = 115g

½ pound = 8 oz = 225g

¾ pound = 12 oz = 340g

1 pound = 16 oz = 454g

Oven Temperature Conversions

200 F = 95 C

250 F = 120 C

275 F = 135 C

300 F = 150 C

325 F = 160 C

350 F = 180 C

375 F = 190 C

400 F = 205 C

425 F = 220 C

450 F = 230 C

Portion Sizes

Portion sizes are a general guide but are based on the

calories given. Appetites are different but if you want to lose weight you must try and stick to the portion size.

Ovens vary so cooking times are only approximate. Always preheat your oven and for fan-assisted ovens reduce the temperature by 20°F or see the manufacturer's instructions for your oven.

Oil - Water Spray

Frying, even shallow frying is not recommended as it can add a lot of calories to any meal. You can make up a solution of 1 part oil to 8 parts water and store it in one of those plastic bottles used as plant demisters that you can get from any store or garden shop.

When you need to grill/broil or dry fry, a few sprays of this solution is enough to lubricate the grill/broiler wire or pan to stop the food sticking. Give the bottle a good shake before using and I recommend sunflower or rapeseed oil. You can even spray the food with this mixture to stop it drying out when you grill/broil or oven bake

BREAKFAST RECIPES

Personally I found it a lot easier not to eat breakfast but this is a matter of choice or your metabolism or your willpower. Some people have to eat breakfast or blood sugar levels drop too much. Try having the porridge made with 50% milk/water with some apple or rhubarb.

If you decide you must have breakfast, there are some delicious shakes or muffins in the book and some tasty cooked breakfasts. You could try to miss lunch altogether and have a more substantial evening meal, although that might be quite hard. If you are struggling to stay within your calorie allowance, don't stress if you go over a little. Just try to remember that a normal calorie intake is 2000 for a woman and 2500 for a man. You are trying to achieve between 500-600 calories for just two days so you **WILL** lose weight even if you go over just a bit.

Simple Breakfasts with Fruit

A typical fasting-day breakfast of 300 calories could be two scrambled eggs with a slice of ham, a good source of protein. But this would only leave you 200 or 300 calories for the rest of the day. Try leaving out the ham and then you would only use 160 calories

Or

Porridge with Raisins and Honey = 224 calories, plenty of water, green tea or black coffee.

Or

1 medium banana, 170g of 0% fat Greek yogurt, 1 tsp of chopped walnuts topped with a tsp of runny honey which is only 150 calories.

Or

Fruit & Yogurt - 140 kcal

140 calories per serving

- Half a small banana
- 170g/ 6oz pot fat free plain yogurt

Just slice banana and add to yogurt

Fruit Fool - 55 kcal

This breakfast recipe can be adapted to seasonal fruits that are easily available in the shops. Choose from any of the following but only use 50g of each.

45- 55 calories per serving
Preparation - 2 minutes

Choose 50g / 2oz of <u>ONE</u> of the following:

- blackberries - fresh peach sliced - raspberries - tinned rhubarb - strawberries
- 50g / 2oz 0% fat Greek yogurt

Mash or chop the chosen fruit and fold into the Greek yogurt.

Fruit Bowl - 100 kcal

You can make a batch of this fruit bowl the night before if you are usually pushed for time in the mornings.

100 - 120 calories per serving
Preparation - 5 minutes

Choose 250g / 9oz of your favourite fruit such as Strawberries, Pink or White Grapefruit, Pineapple, Raspberries, Peaches or Nectarines, Kiwi Fruit. **<u>No Banana though.</u>**

Method
Prepare and mix together your chosen fruits and then just weigh out 250 grams for breakfast on your fasting days. You can snack on the surplus on your other days if you like or save for your second day as it will keep in the fridge just fine

SMOOTHIES

Breakfast Smoothies are very healthy and a great alternative to grabbing that really unhealthy breakfast on your way to work or when you take the kids to school.

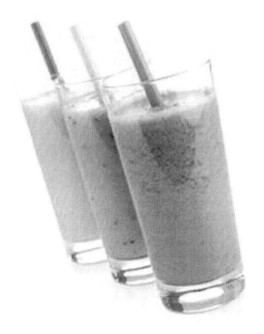

Banana & Berry - 94 kcal

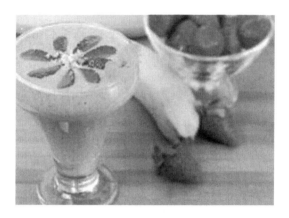

94 calories per serving
Preparation - 5 minutes

Ingredients

- ½ banana
- 50g / 1¾ oz / ¼ cup frozen or fresh strawberries
- 25g / 1 oz / ¼ cup frozen or fresh blueberries
- ¼ cup flavoured water (no sugar added)

Method

If using frozen fruit let it sit out a little bit, perhaps as you shower etc. When they have thawed slightly, add all ingredients in the blender. Add a little extra water if you have trouble blending the frozen fruit.

When the consistency is almost sorbet like, your smoothie is done. Scrumptious!!

Spinach - 85 kcal

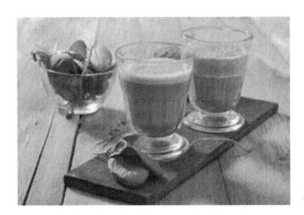

A healthy green smoothie, a perfect way to kick start the day.

85 calories per serving
Preparation - 5 minutes

Ingredients
*   10g / ⅓ cup raw spinach
*   35g / 1¼ cup pineapple chunks
*   1 oz non-fat strawberry banana yogurt
*   ½ small banana
*   40g / 1½ fl oz / filtered water

Method
Mix everything in the blender until smooth and then just serve.

Strawberry & Banana - 75 kcal

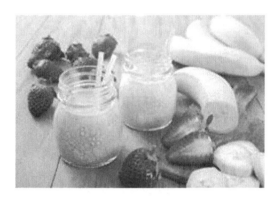

Another non-fat smoothie to get your fasting day going and keep you on track.

75 calories per serving
Preparation - 5 minutes

Ingredients

- 60ml / 2 fl oz / ¼ cup non-fat yogurt
- ½ small banana
- 2 large strawberries

Method

Simply slice the strawberries and banana, add to blender and whizz till well combined.

Strawberry Kiwi - 85 kcal

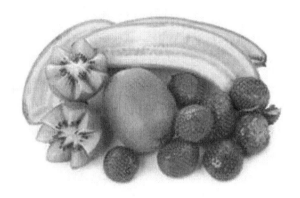

85 calories per serving
Preparation - 5 minutes

Ingredients

- 75 ml / 2½ fl oz / ⅓ cup cold apple juice
- ½ ripe banana, peeled
- ½ ripe kiwi peeled and sliced
- 250g / 9 oz / 1¼ cups fresh or frozen strawberries
- ½ tsp honey

Method

Put everything into a blender, and combine until smooth.

Watermelon Juice - 33 kcal

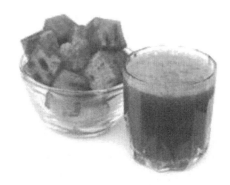

Very low calorie, very refreshing drink, especially if you take it along with you when you exercise in the mornings.

33 calories per serving
Preparation - 5 minutes

Ingredients

- 110 g watermelon
- 15 ice cubes water

Method

Place seedless watermelon and ice cubes in blender. For an extra bit of energy, add some sugar free Red Bull or any other diet soda. Blend until desired result.

Pack into water bottle and enjoy your morning exercise or work journey.

Fruits & Honey - 160 kcal

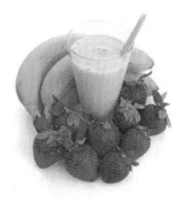

An amazing smoothie packed full of goodness and very quick to prepare.

160 calories per serving
Preparation - 2 minutes

Ingredients

- 100g / 3½ oz / ½ cup frozen or fresh strawberries
- 2 tsp honey
- ½ banana
- ½ tsp vanilla essence/extract
- 125ml / 4 fl oz / ½ cup fat free milk

Method

Prepare and blend all ingredients together in a blender until smooth. Add seven large ice cubes if using fresh rather than frozen fruit.

Breakfast Smoothie - 175 kcal

A high protein as well as a low fat tasty breakfast smoothie with an unusual ingredient.

185 calories per serving
Preparation - 5 minutes

Ingredients

- ¼ tsp vanilla essence/extract
- ½ small banana
- 25g / 1oz / ¼ cup blueberries fresh or frozen
- 25ml / 1 fl oz / ¼ cup orange juice
- 30g / 1oz / 1 cup baby spinach, chopped
- 1 oz soya protein powder
- ½ packet (½ serving) sugar substitute (like Splenda)

Method

In a blender mix juice with the berries, add banana and spinach and mix. Add protein powder and sugar substitute and blend again.

Enjoy!

Note: try different frozen fruit, just check calorie count.

Chocolate Soya Milk Shake - 165 kcal

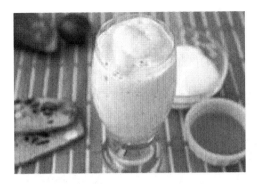

A soya milk shake that has a bit of a kick in it.

165 calories per serving
Preparation - 5 minutes

Ingredients

- 225g / 4 oz / ½ cup low fat cottage cheese
- 1 good helping ice
- 125ml / 4 fl oz / ½ cup vanilla soya milk
- 1 tbsp unsweetened cocoa
- 2 servings 1 packet sweetener (like Splenda)

Method

Simply put everything into a blender and mix on high setting until ice is broken down and blended well.

Green Juice - 175 kcal

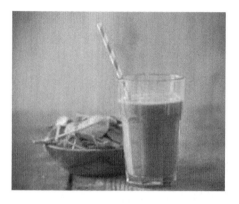

Fruits and vegetables juice really well together and are ideal with some ice when it's hot outside.

175 calories per serving
Preparation - 5 minutes

Ingredients

- 15g / ½ oz / ½ cup baby spinach
- 5 mint leaves
- 50ml / 2 fl oz / ¼ cup lemon juice
- 200g / 7 oz / 1 cup diced pineapple
- 150g / 5 oz / 1 cup cucumber

Method

Put the pineapple and the cucumber into the blender and mix a little. Add the other ingredients and blend together. Add some crushed ice to freshen.

Kombucha Ginger - 120 kcal

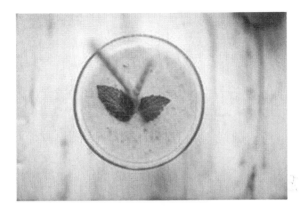

This smoothie uses green tea called Kombucha which is readily available in most health shops and some larger food markets. I have used the ginger flavoured one but you will have your favourite.

120 calories per serving
Preparation - 10 minutes

Ingredients

- ½ small cucumber, chopped
- 1 ripe kiwi, peeled
- 125ml / 4 fl oz / ½ cup ginger-flavoured Kombucha green tea
- 60g / 2oz / ¼ cup low-fat plain Greek yogurt
- 1 tablespoons fresh coriander / cilantro leaves
- 4 ice cubes

Combine all ingredients in a blender until smooth.

Orange & Veggie - 180 kcal

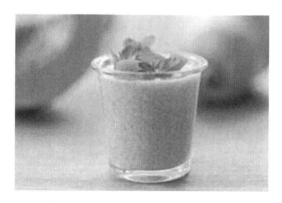

A quick and simple smoothie to have when in a rush.
Ingredients look dull but it really does taste great and so
healthy!

180 calories per serving
Preparation - 3 minutes

Ingredients

- ½ large banana
- 225ml / 8 fl oz / 1 cup orange juice
- 15g / ½ oz / ½ cup fresh spinach

Method

Put all ingredients in blender and blend on slow for
30 seconds so that it doesn't froth up too much.

Very Quick Smoothie - 170 kcal

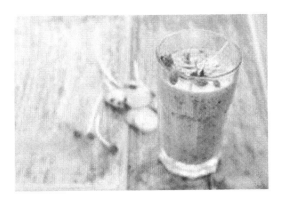

Here is a very quick and simple way to make a smoothie for breakfast so you can start your day off right. You could even mix it in a travel mug so you can take it with you in the car.

170 calories per serving
Preparation - 1 minute

Ingredients

- 125ml / 4 fl oz / ½ cup low fat milk
- 125ml / 4 fl oz / ½ cup low fat fruit yogurt

Mix half a container of your favourite low fat/low calorie fruit yogurt with half a cup of milk.

Try substituting light soy-milk for extra protein.

Strawberry Protein Flax - 145 kcal

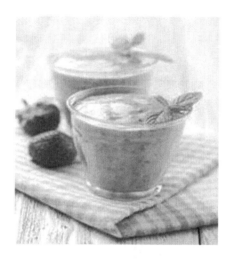

This makes a good protein rich breakfast for a busy morning and you can also have it for a healthy snack at any other time of the day.

145 calories per serving
Preparation - 15 minutes

Ingredients

- 150g / 5 oz / ¾ cup fresh or frozen strawberries
- 1 tsp ground flax seed
- 50ml / 2 fl oz / ¼ cup unsweetened vanilla almond milk
- 25ml / 2 fl oz / ⅛ cup non fat vanilla Greek yogurt
- 20g / ¾ oz granulated sugar

Method

Pour all ingredients into blender in the following order - milk, flax, sugar, yogurt, strawberries and then 2 cups of ice cubes.

Blend on high speed until completely smooth and serve with a sprig of mint on top.

Wide Awake Smoothie
- 140 kcal

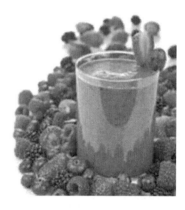

If you keep a good supply of frozen fruit in your freezer you will always have a delicious smoothie to kick-start your fasting day.

140 calories per serving
preparation - 5 minutes

Ingredients

- 90ml / 3½ fl oz fresh orange juice
- ½ medium banana
- 55g / 1½ oz ½ cup frozen berries, such as raspberries, blackberries, blueberries, strawberries
- 40g / 1½ oz low-fat plain yogurt
- 1 tsp sugar or sugar substitute

Method

Place all ingredients in a blender and mix until smooth.

Notes

COOKED BREAKFASTS

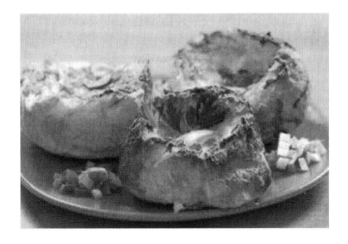

Easy Fry Up - 195 kcal

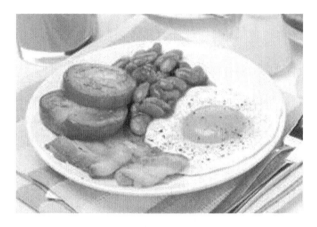

This breakfast includes a portion of baked beans which will make it quite filling.

195 calories per serving
Cooking - 5 minutes

Ingredients

- · 1 reduced fat bacon rasher
- · 1 large egg
- 2 slices tomato
- · 100g / 4oz reduced sugar and salt baked beans

Method

Heat a small non stick frying pan on a medium heat and when hot, add the bacon to the pan.

Fry for about 1 minute before turning over and then add the egg.

Fry until the egg is cooked to your liking. In the meantime heat the baked beans in a small saucepan or better still microwave covered for 1 minute. Serve with the egg and bacon and enjoy.

Corn & Onion Bake - 110 kcal

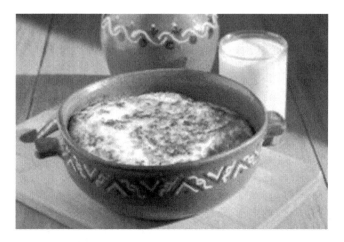

A really easy baked omelette with onions and corn. You can substitute any green vegetable if you don't like corn, just check the calorie count.

110 calories per serving
Preparation - 10 minutes
Cooking - 30 minutes

Ingredients

- 125ml / 4 fl oz / ½ cup egg whites
- ½ tsp garlic powder
- ½ tsp paprika
- 40g / 1½ oz / ¼ cup cooked sweetcorn
- 1 medium spring onion / scallion

Method

Preheat oven to 350 °F (175 °C)

Chop the onion very finely. Mix together the egg whites, corn and onions in a bowl. Add the salt, pepper, paprika and garlic power.

Spray a small baking pan with low calorie spray or your oil and water mixture. Pour all of the ingredients into the pan and bake until brown on top.

*****You can find ready prepared egg whites in most large food stores and they keep well in the fridge for use in other fasting day meals. They come in milk like cartons and are very low calorie.

***A 500g carton of egg white contains the equivalent of 15 eggs, so the recipe above would need about 3-4 eggs, which is quite a lot of yolks to use up, so try to get the ready prepared if you can.

Egg & Bacon Roll - 196 kcal

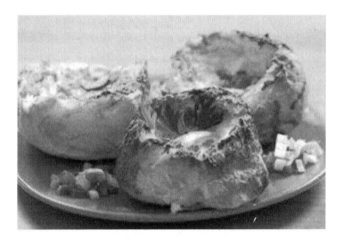

This is so simple to make it is almost a cheek putting in as a recipe but it would be a shame if you missed out on one of these, they are delicious.

I have given ingredients for 1 but as you can see each roll is made individually but can be made in bigger batches for perhaps a family breakfast. Just remember though, you can only have one.

196 calories per serving
Preparation - 5 minutes
Cooking - 25 minutes

Ingredients

- 1 thin slice of bacon chopped
- 1 large egg
- 1 tbsp grated parmesan cheese

- 1 bread roll

Method

Preheat the oven to 350° F (175° C).

Slice off the tops of the bread rolls about ½ inch deep and scoop out the inner dough so that you can fill them.

Crack an egg into each hollowed out roll and add the bacon pieces on top. Finish off with a third of the grated cheese on each roll.

Place on a baking tin/sheet in the middle of the preheated oven and bake for 20 minutes.

Pop the bread tops back on the baked rolls and cook for an additional 5 minutes

Egg White French Toast - 80 kcal

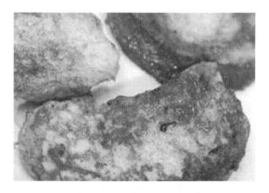

Yummy, Yummy, Yummy, I'll say no more.

80 calories per serving
Preparation - 2 minutes
Cooking - 3-5 minutes

Ingredients

- 1 slice of bread
- 2 tbsp fat free milk
- 1 medium egg (white only)
- ⅛ tsp or a few drops of vanilla essence/extract
- pinch of cinnamon

Method

Preheat your non stick frying pan/skillet on a medium heat.

Separate the egg and mix together the egg white, fat free milk, vanilla, and cinnamon in a small bowl.

Pour onto a flat dinner plate and soak each side of your slice of bread in the egg mixture.

Heat a frying pan or skillet and spray with a low cal oil spray. Cook on both sides making sure you flip to avoid burning. When both sides are brown and firm it is ready.

Enjoy!

Egg & Cheese Sandwich - 95 kcal

This is just a bit of treat for breakfast and is quite satisfying and filling.

95 calories per serving
Preparation - 2 minutes
Cooking - 5 minutes

Ingredients

- 1 large egg white*****
- 1 slice of Kraft fat free cheese (Kraft singles)
- 1 slice of toast
- ¼ tsp water

Method

Beat the egg white and water together and season to taste.

Heat a small non stick fry pan / skillet and cook egg as normal.

Toast your bread as the egg white cooks. When your egg white is done place the slice of cheese on top of the egg and let it melt.

Cut the slice of toast in half and make a sandwich with the cooked egg and cheese.

*****You can find ready prepared egg whites in most large food stores and they keep well in the fridge for use in other fasting day meals. They come in milk like cartons and are very low calorie.

A 500g carton of egg white contains the equivalent of 15 eggs, so the recipe above would need about 35g.

Egg White Omelette - 60 kcal

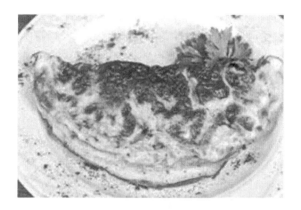

60 calories per serving
Preparation - 2 minutes
Cooking - 2 minutes

Ingredients

- 3 large eggs
- a few basil or other fresh herb leaves
- 3 sprays light sunflower oil

Method

Separate the eggs and save the yolks for a non fasting day meal.

Whisk together the egg whites and a good helping of salt and pepper. Spray the oil into a non stick pan and heat until the pan looks hot. Pour in the egg whites and cook until ready but not too dry.

Serve at once with the herb leaves and a sprinkling of paprika if liked.

*****You can find ready prepared egg whites in most large food stores and they keep well in the fridge for use in other fasting day meals. They come in milk like cartons and are very low calorie.

A 500g carton of egg white contains the equivalent of 15 eggs, so the recipe above would need about 100g.

Omelette & Tomatoes - 147 kcal

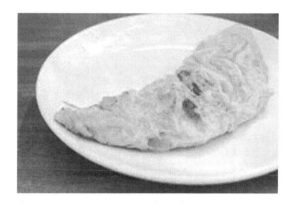

Just a simple omelette using egg whites and fresh tomatoes.

147 calories per serving
Preparation - 1 minute
Cooking - 5 minutes

Ingredients

- 6 large egg whites*****
- 1 tsp hot chilli sauce
- 2 medium tomatoes, any type

Method

Beat the eggs whites and fry in a non-stick/Teflon pan.

Chop up the tomatoes and add half to the pan.

When the omelette is ready, put on a warmed plate and serve the remaining tomato on top.

Season with the hot chilli sauce and salt and pepper to taste.

You can serve almost anything with this omelette, try a few mushrooms lightly sautéed or some chopped spring onions/scallions.

***You can find ready prepared egg whites in most large food stores and they keep well in the fridge for use in other fasting day meals. They come in milk like cartons and are very low calorie.

A 500g carton of egg white contains the equivalent of 15 eggs, so the recipe above would need about 200g.

Ham & Eggs - 190 kcal

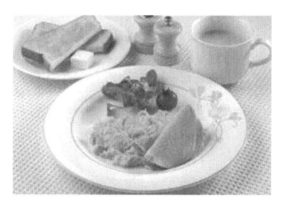

A variation on scrambled eggs that is both filling and very quick to do

190 calories per serving
Preparation - 5 minutes
Cooking - 10 minutes

Ingredients

- ¼ any bell pepper, chopped
- 1 large egg
- 1 large egg white
- 1 oz extra lean sliced ham, chopped
- 25g / 1 oz / ¼ cup mushroom pieces
- 35g / 1¼ oz / ¼ cup onions, chopped

Method

Spray small non stick frying pan / skillet with low cal spray oil or oil and water spray.

Add the vegetables and ham to the pan and cook until soft but not burnt.

Add the egg and egg white, stir through and carry on cooking until eggs are firm.

Season to taste and serve hot.

Kippers - 125 kcal

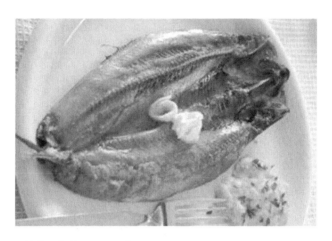

125 calories per serving
Preparation – 2 minutes
Cooking – 2-3 minutes

There are roughly 125 calories in an average sized smoked kipper fillet, so this will make a quick and satisfying breakfast.

Either cook as normal under the grill or for a no smell method, place in a suitable dish with a wedge of lemon, add a tbsp milk, cover with cling wrap and microwave for two and a half minutes and voila, tasty breakfast that hasn't used up too much of your allowance.

Low Cal Fried Breakfast - 178 kcal

This is a bit of a cheats fry up but when you really fancy something a bit tastier on one of your fasting days then this will hit the spot. Most supermarkets have the medallion type bacon usually classed as reduced fat. If not, just cut off the tail of the bacon and all of the fat.

178 calories per serving
Cooking- 10 minutes

Ingredients

- 2 reduced fat bacon rashers
- 1 large egg
- 1 medium tomato halved

Method

Heat a non stick frying pan until hot. Add the bacon and when it starts to release some fat or liquid, swish it around the pan to coat and then add the two tomato halves. Fry for about 2 minutes or until they are both starting to brown.

Turn the bacon and tomatoes over and move to one side of the pan. Crack the egg into the space and fry for another three minutes. If the egg is not fully cooked, pop a lid or splash guard on top to help it along and then just serve.

Mushroom & Spinach Bake - 86 kcal

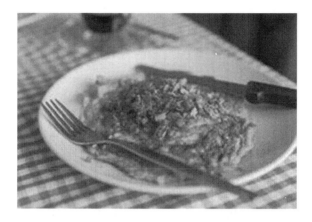

This is a very quick dish to do and looks a little like a mini pizza.

86 calories per serving
Preparation - 10 minutes
Cooking - 20 minutes

Ingredients

- ½ oz mozzarella cheese
- ½ tsp garlic powder
- 1 large portabella flat mushroom
- 8- 10 spinach leaves

Method

Preheat oven to 375 °F (190 °C).

Clean and cut off the stem from the Portabella mushroom.

Wash the spinach leaves and dry as much water off as you can. Fill the inside of the mushroom cap with the spinach and the chopped up stem. Sprinkle the cheese on top of the mushroom, then the powdered garlic and seasoned salt.

Place filled mushroom cap onto a baking sheet. Cook for 12 to 16 minutes or until cheese is melted.

Porridge Oats with Fruit - 136 kcal

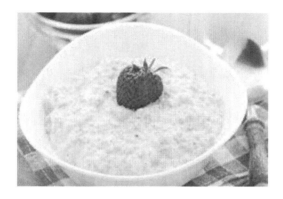

136 calories per serving
Preparation - 2 minutes
Cooking - 3 minutes

Ingredients

- 30g / 1¼ oz uncooked porridge oats
- 200ml / 7 fl oz / 1 scant cup of skimmed milk and water mixed 50/50
- 50g / 2oz strawberries or 2 tbsp of stewed plums or rhubarb or half a banana
- A dribble of honey if needed but try to do without.

Method

In a large 3.5 pint jug or bowl, mix porridge oats with the milk or 50/50 mix and microwave on high for 2 minutes, stir and microwave for a further minute, serve topped with one of the above fruits and the honey.

Simple Poached Eggs - 145 kcal

This has got to be the quickest breakfast you can do if you are really pushed for time as it is done in the microwave, so no mess either.

145 calories per serving
Preparation - 1 minute
Cooking - 2 minutes

Ingredients

- low calorie cooking spray
- 2 large eggs

Method

Spray a small microwavable bowl with a low calorie cooking spray or oil & water spray. Make sure you completely coat the whole bowl.

Break both eggs into bowl and pierce egg yolks with a fork or similar.

Spray eggs with cooking spray and season with salt and pepper (optional.)

Cover bowl with a spatter-proof lid and microwave on high for 1½ minutes for softer yolks or 2 minutes for harder set yolks.

Serve with half a slice of toast, a handful of cress or parsley.

Salsa Eggs - 125 kcal

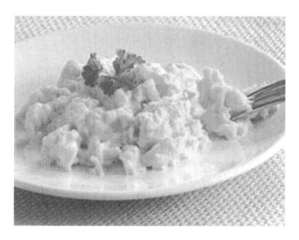

One of my favourite breakfast egg recipes, yummy and simple.

125 calories per serving
Preparation - 1 minute
Cooking - 3 minutes

Ingredients

- 4 large egg whites (see below)
- 1 tsp paprika
- 1 tsp black pepper
- 1 tbsp salsa
- ½ medium whole tomato, chopped

Method

Beat the egg whites together with salt and pepper to taste. Cook in a frying pan/skillet over medium heat.

When the eggs are cooked to your liking, serve on a plate with the chopped tomatoes on top and the paprika and salsa sprinkled all over.

*****You can find ready prepared egg whites in most large food stores and they keep well in the fridge for use in other fasting day meals. They come in milk like cartons and are very low calorie.*

A 500g carton of egg white contains the equivalent of 15 eggs, so the recipe above would need about 130g.

Scrambled Eggs Various - 170 kcal

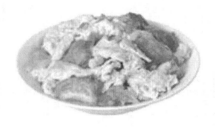

170 calories per serving
Preparation - 2 minutes
Cooking - 3 minutes

Ingredients

- 2 medium eggs
- 1 medium tomato
- 1 tsp of fresh herbs to taste
- pinch of chilli flakes (optional)

Method

Chop the tomato and microwave with the chilli flakes (optional) for about 45 seconds to heat. Do your scrambled eggs how you like them but preferably not overcooked and just add the heated tomato at the end to serve.

You can also replace the tomato with either 100g mushrooms or 100g spring onions. Just slice and fry off in a small non stick pan, with just a spray of oil and add to the scrambled egg.

This may not be satisfying for everyone, but if you really need to eat something rather than go without breakfast, then this makes a change from porridge.

Soya Protein Pancake - 95 kcal

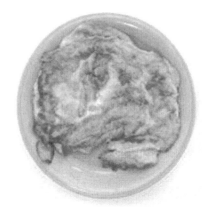

This makes good use of soya protein which is available in most health shops or big food stores and is so easy to make you don't need to make bigger batches.

95 calories per serving
Preparation - 2 minutes
Cooking - 5 minutes

Ingredients

- 3 fl oz water
- 1 oz soy/soya protein

Method

Simply mix the protein powder and water to a pancake batter like consistency.

Spray a small pancake pan or griddle and heat until hot.

Cook the pancake slowly, trying not to dry it out in the middle too much.

Serve with a sprinkling of cinnamon or honey to taste.

Tomato & Onion Omelette - 180 kcal

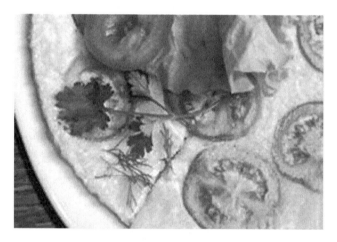

A very simple filling omelette, ideal for a quick breakfast.

180 calories per serving
Preparation - 3-5 minutes
Cooking - 5-8 minutes

Ingredients

- 2 eggs
- dash of skimmed milk
- 1 tomato chopped
- 2 spring onions / scallions sliced

Method

Spray a small omelette pan / skillet with low cal spray or oil and water spray.

Fry the chopped tomato and spring onions until soft then add beaten eggs and milk. Stir very slightly so vegetables are covered and cook until firm.

Notes

EASY LUNCHES

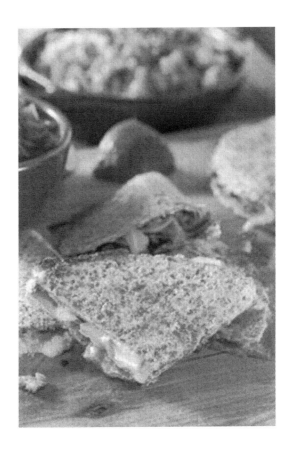

BLT Sandwich - 175 kcal

This is a quick but satisfying lunch and you can have it because it uses low fat bacon

175 calories per serving
Preparation - 2 minutes
Cooking - 5 minutes

Ingredients

- 1 low calorie flatbread or 100 cal 'Thin' roll
- 1 low fat bacon rasher
- 1 tsp lighter salad cream
- 1 medium tomato
- lettuce

Method

Grill or dry fry the bacon and drain off any liquid or fat. Lightly toast the flatbread and build the sandwich by spreading the salad cream over the flatbread, top with the sliced lettuce and then bacon rasher and finally add the sliced tomato.

Cottage Cheese & Various - 109 kcal

109 calories per serving plus

Choose from the following

Ingredients

- 1xKallo Organic Rice Cakes – 30 kcal
- 1xRyvita Crackers for Cheese – 27 kcal
- 1xJacobs Choice Grain Cracker – 33 kcal
- 100g Reduced Fat Cottage Cheese

Method

Just choose the biscuit you would like to put your cottage cheese on and calculate how many you can eat within you daily allowance.

Top with a sliver of cucumber or tomato, salt and pepper.

Poached Eggs & Spinach - 200 kcal

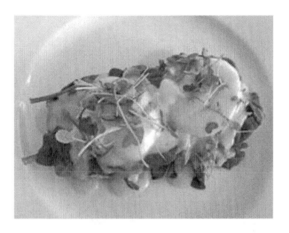

200 calories per serving
Preparation - 5 minutes
Cooking - 10 minutes

Ingredients

- 1 bag fresh spinach
- 2 eggs

Method

Poach the eggs as you like them. I find those silicone poaching pods are great and always deliver a perfect egg.

Rinse the spinach in a colander or sieve and pour a kettle of boiling water over it to wilt.

Drain off excess water by pressing into the colander or sieve with a potato masher or other flat tool.

Place on warmed plate and top with poached eggs, a sprinkling of spinach leaves and season to taste.

You can use frozen spinach if more convenient, just defrost 200g naturally, squeeze excess water out and heat gently until warmed through.

Potato Salad - 120 kcal

120 calories per serving
Preparation - 10 minutes
Cooking – 20 minutes

Ingredients

- 125g / 4½ oz small or new potatoes
- 1 tbsp low-fat salad cream (20 cals)
- 1 tbsp low-fat Greek yoghurt
- ½ tsp Dijon mustard
- 6 spring onions
- ¼ of a cucumber

Method

Cut the potatoes into roughly 2cm chunks and bring to the boil in a pan of lightly salted water and cook for 10-15 minutes or until soft.

Mix together the low-fat salad cream and yogurt add the mustard and mix it in well.

Drain the potatoes and put them in a large bowl. When they have cooled a little, stir in the mayonnaise mixture and leave to cool completely.

Chop the spring onions and cucumber and add them to the cold potato salad, mix well, season to taste and serve.

This potato salad can be made in bigger batches and served at lunch or dinner with your other chosen foods.

At 120 calories a serving it makes a nice lunch with half a tin of tuna in water drained (70cals) and a chopped tomato (10cals).

If you prefer mayonnaise add anoth 50 calories per serving.

Tuna Salad -106 kcal

106 calories per serving
Preparation – 10 minutes

Ingredients

- 1 tomato
- 2 sticks celery
- 5 thick slices of cucumber,
- 1 spring onion
- ½ tin of tuna in spring water drained
- 1 tbsp of low-fat salad cream (20 cals).

Method

Chop or slice all salad ingredients to your taste. Stir salad cream into the Tuna and mix into the prepared salad. (You can keep the other half in the fridge and use for your next fasting day lunch or use it for a sandwich on a non fasting day.)

You can use mayonnaise if preferred but add another 50 calories. Drizzle over a little balsamic glaze and a few basil leaves if you have them for extra flavour.

LESS THAN 200 CALORIES VEGETARIAN

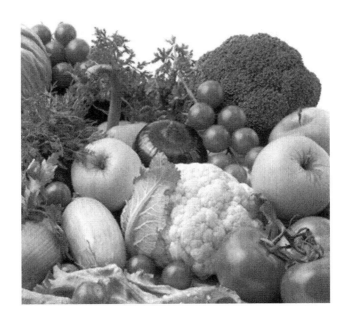

Butternut Squash Soup - 200 kcal

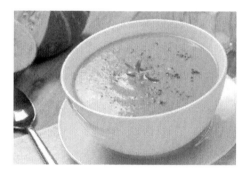

This is a thick and warming soup that is delicious on a cold day. Make bigger batches and freeze.

200 calories per serving
***Suitable for freezing
Preparation - 10-15 minutes
Cooking - 25-30 minutes

Ingredients

- ½ tsp olive oil
- ½ small onion, chopped
- 1 clove of garlic, chopped
- portion of butternut squash – about 125g / 4½ oz
- 225ml / 8 fl oz / 1 cup of vegetable stock
- 1 pinch cayenne pepper

Method

Heat the oil in a large pan. Add the onion and garlic and cook very gently for about 5 minutes until translucent and sticky but not burnt.

Prepare the squash by cutting into quarters; take out the seeds and then peel. Cut the remaining flesh into small chunks and when onion is ready, add the squash to the pan.

Stir, add the stock and cayenne pepper and bring to a low simmer. Lower the heat and cook for about 20 minutes. When squash is ready, leave to cool slightly and either use a blender or mash it by hand. Season to taste, add a little more hot stock or water if the soup is too thick.

Easy Mixed Salad - 40 kcal

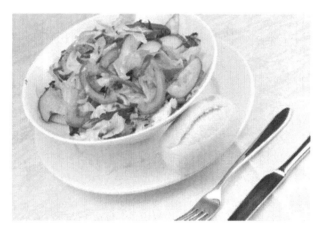

You can have this salad with any of your chosen meats or fish for lunch or dinner. It is a staple of my fasting days and I will eat this for lunch with ½ can tuna in spring water, drained and mixed with a tbsp of low calorie salad cream. I also have this with an omelette either hot or cold on my non-fasting days because it is easy to make and very good to eat and keeps me off the bread and cakes.

40 calories per serving
Preparation 5-10 minutes

Ingredients

- 1 tomato
- 2 sticks celery
- 6 thick slices of cucumber,

- 2 spring onions/scallions
- 1 tbsp of reduced fat salad cream (20cal)
- Squeeze of balsamic glaze

Method

If you prefer, peel the celery. Chop or slice all salad ingredients. Stir salad cream into the prepared salad.

You can use mayonnaise if preferred but add another 50 calories. I have tried the low calorie mayonnaise but because they have taken oil out to reduce the calories it is quite tasteless and dry. I much prefer salad cream, it has a lot more bite.

Drizzle over a little balsamic glaze for a bit more flavour.

Hearty Potato & Leek Soup - 150 kcal

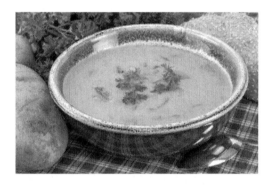

This soup is so delicious, you really should make bigger batches of it and freeze for convenience.

150 calories per serving
***Suitable for freezing
Preparation - 15 minutes
Cooking - 45 minutes

Ingredients

- 250g/8oz small leeks, untrimmed
- 100g / 3½ oz potatoes
- 1 cal oil spray
- 100g / 3½ oz button mushrooms
- A few sprigs of Tarragon, stalks removed
- 80ml / 3 fl oz / ⅓ cup of skimmed milk

Method

Trim the leeks, cut into thin slices and place in cold water to get rid of any soil.

Peel and cut the potatoes into 2cm cubes. Heat 5 pumps of the oil spray in a large pan over a medium heat.

Thoroughly drain the leeks and add to the pan. Cook gently for about 5 minutes. Add the potatoes and tarragon leaves and enough water to cover. Cook the vegetables for 15-20 minutes with the lid on, then add the milk and the sliced mushrooms and cook for another 20 minutes, adding more water if necessary.

Take out about ¼ of the soup including some potatoes and mash or whiz smooth. Return to the pan, season to taste and serve hot.

Lentil & Greens Soup - 140 kcal

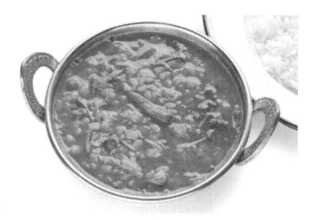

The lentils and greens make a colourful combination and the taste is not bad either. Alternate the choice of greens and spinach for variety.

140 calories per serving
Preparation - 10 minutes
Cooking 30-35 minutes

Ingredients

- 50g / 2 oz green lentils
- 1 small onion
- 1 cloves of garlic
- 1 cal oil spray
- 50g / 2 oz fresh spring greens or spinach
- 200ml / 7oz / 1 cup of vegetable stock or water

Method

Rinse the lentils under running water and cook them in fresh water for 10-15 minutes until just beginning to go soft. Drain and rinse again.

Peel and chop the onion and garlic. Put 5 pumps of the oil in a large pan and cook the onion until soft but not burnt, then add the garlic and lentils.

Wash and chop the greens or spinach and add it to the pan gradually, allowing it to shrink down but keep stirring.

When all the greens or spinach are in, reduce it by about half, add enough liquid to cover and cook for about 15 minutes if spring greens, 10 minutes if using spinach.

Allow to cool slightly, blend, reheat and serve.

Low Calorie Hummus - 125 kcal

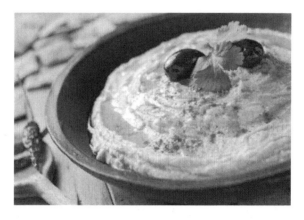

Hummus is a great little snacking or lunch food. It is quite filling if you have 3 rice cakes at 30 calories each with a thin slice of cucumber or tomato on top.

125 calories per serving
Preparation 5-10 minutes
Cooking 5 minutes

Ingredients

- 100g / 3½ oz of cooked chickpeas (canned or fresh)
- 1 clove of garlic
- juice of ½ lemon
- 1 tsp tahini paste

Method

Drain and rinse the chickpeas if using canned or cook the dried chickpeas as per instructions on packet.

Put in a pan and cover with a little fresh water and heat gently for about 5 minutes. Drain the chickpeas but keep some of the liquid and set aside.

Crush the garlic, place in a food processor with the chickpeas and lemon juice. Add the tahini and a tablespoon of the cooking liquid and process until smooth, adding more liquid if necessary.

For dipping

½ red pepper, de-seeded and sliced into batons
2 inches cucumber, cut into batons
½ carrot, peeled and cut into batons

Mixed Salad & Avocado - 120 kcal

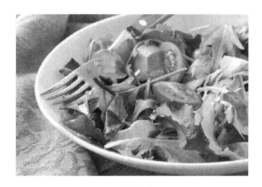

A simple salad that goes with anything. Try it on its own for lunch or with a salmon or Tuna steak for your evening meal.

120 calories per serving
Preparation - 5 minutes

Ingredients

- 60- 80gm bag mixed salad leaves or rocket
- 3 small tomatoes
- 1 small or half a medium ripe avocado
- Selection of fresh herbs such as basil, mint or chives (optional)
- Olive oil and balsamic vinegar for drizzling

Method

Slice or quarter the tomatoes, wash and shred the mixed salad. Mix with the herbs if using and place in a good sized bowl.

Peel and slice the avocado, lay on top of the salad and drizzle with the dressing.

Pea & Spinach Dahl - 170 kcal

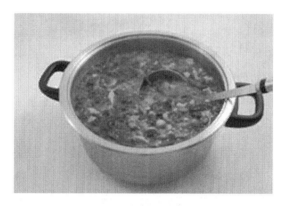

This dish will warm and fill you up on your fasting day, what more could you want?

170 calories per serving
***Suitable for freezing
Preparation - 10 minutes
Cooking - 50 minutes

Ingredients

- 1 small onion
- 1 clove garlic
- 1 thumb size piece fresh ginger
- 1 small red chilli
- 1 cal oil spray
- 50g / 2oz red lentils
- ¼ tsp of both turmeric powder and cayenne pepper

- ¼ tsp paprika
- ¼ tsp ground cumin
- 300ml / ½ pint water
- 1 small tomato
- juice of ½ lime
- 1 tbsp frozen peas
- 1 cube frozen spinach

Method

Peel and roughly chop the onion, garlic and ginger. Do the same to the chilli but if you don't want it too hot you can remove all or some of the seeds.

Heat 5 pumps of the oil in a heavy based pan and sauté all chopped ingredients for about 5 minutes or until the onion has softened. Add all the ground spices and fry for another couple of minutes stirring well.

Rinse the lentils in a sieve under cold running water for at least a minute and add them to the pan. Stir really well and then add the water and bring back to a boil. Boil at a steady rate for 10 minutes and then turn the heat down to a low simmer.

Continue to simmer at the lowest heat for about 30 to 40 minutes, making sure you stir the Dahl often to stop it sticking on the bottom of the pan. The mixture will thicken as it cooks and when it looks like thick rice pudding, add the spinach, peas, lime juice and the chopped tomato and cook for another 5 minutes and then serve in warmed bowls.

Ratatouille - 105 kcal

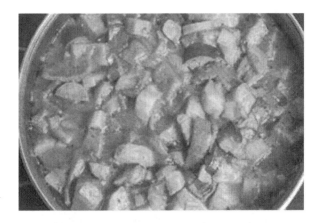

This dish can be served with any fish or meat for a substantial evening meal as the ratatouille is only 105 calories per serving. You can have a lean pork steak or grilled chicken breast or salmon fillet or any other meat or fish choice. You could even have a medium jacket potato which is 136 calories per 100g. Just check the weight when choosing. You could add it to a couple of eggs and make a tasty crepe for lunch or supper.

105 calories per serving for the ratatouille
Preparation - 10-15 minutes
Cooking - 20 minutes plus time to cook chosen
   meat/fish

Ingredients

- 1 small onion
- 1 garlic clove
- ½ small green bell pepper
- ½ small yellow bell pepper
- 1 small courgette
- 50g / 2oz button mushrooms
- 200g / 7oz can chopped tomatoes
- 1 tbsp tomato paste
- ½ tsp of dried mixed herbs

Method

Peel and chop the onion, trim, deseed and dice both peppers and the courgette. Halve and chop the mushrooms, chop the garlic.

Put all vegetables into a pan and add the chopped tomatoes and tomato paste and stir well. Add the dried herbs, a tsp of sugar and plenty of seasoning. Bring to the boil and simmer uncovered for 20 minutes.

Tomato & Pepper Soup - 120 kcal

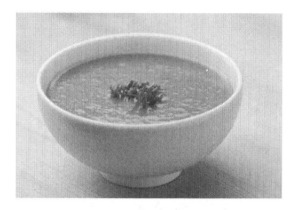

This makes a great starter or a light lunch and is very easy to make. Make bigger batches for freezing.

120 calories per serving
***Suitable for freezing
Preparation - 10 minutes
Cooking - 30 minutes

Ingredients

- ½ red pepper
- 1 garlic cloves
- 1 small onion
- ½ tsp olive oil
- 200g / 7oz tin of chopped tomatoes
- 20g / 1oz potatoes

Method

De-seed and chop the peppers into chunks. Chop or dice the onion and the garlic. Peel and cut the potatoes into good sized chunks and keep in water until needed.

Heat a pan over a medium heat and when warm, add the peppers, onion and garlic and allow them to cook for about 5 minutes until softened. Make sure you stir often so that they don't stick. Add the tinned tomatoes and potatoes and using the tomato can as a measure add ½ can of water to cover.

Simmer the soup for about 20 minutes until the vegetables are done, then allow them to cool slightly and blend until smooth. Reheat and serve.

This makes 4 portions but can be frozen for another fasting day

Tzatsiki - 50 kcal

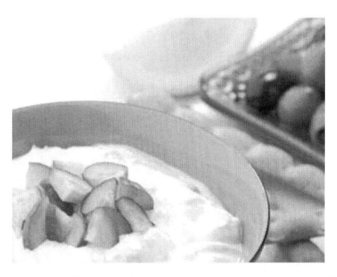

A versatile and quick to prepare dip or salsa that will go with most fish and meat dishes or any salads.

50 calories per serving
Preparation - 10 minutes

Ingredients

- ¼ medium cucumber
- 1 cloves of garlic
- a handful of flat-leaved parsley or coriander
- a few mint leaves
- 50ml / 1½oz / ¼ cup low-fat Greek yogurt
- ½ tsp olive oil
- cayenne and black pepper

Method

Cut the cucumber in half across, and then cut each part in half lengthwise. Remove the seeds and chop the cucumber finely.

Chop the herbs and garlic and put them in a bowl, then add the cucumber. Stir everything together really well.

Add the yogurt and again mix well. Drizzle the olive oil on top and sprinkle with half tsp cayenne and some freshly ground black pepper.

Vegetable Curry- 185 kcal

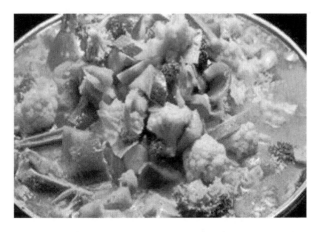

You could use a pre-mixed madras curry powder instead of the spices. This could also be made in bigger portions and frozen. You could also use fresh vegetables; adjust the cooking time to make sure they are cooked before serving the curry.

185 calories per serving
***Suitable for freezing
Preparation 5 minutes
Cooking 40 minutes

Ingredients

- 1 tsp sunflower oil
- ½ tsp each of cumin seeds and mustard seeds
- ½ onion
- 1 clove garlic

- ¼ tsp ground coriander, cumin and turmeric
- ½ tsp mild chilli powder
- ½ tsp salt
- ½ tin chopped tomatoes
- 2 good handfuls of pre-chopped frozen vegetables (choose from carrot, peas, green beans, cauliflower, or anything else you like!)

Method

Finely chop the onion and garlic. Heat the oil and cook the cumin and mustard seeds until the spices start to pop but do not burn them.

Add the chopped onion and garlic, stir and lower the heat to a simmer. Cook the onions for about 10 minutes until they are translucent and starting to go brown.

Add the remaining spices and salt, stir thoroughly and then put in the chopped tomatoes.

Add your choice of vegetables, bring back to the boil and then simmer gently for 15 minutes adding a little water if mixture starts to dry out.

Notes

FISH

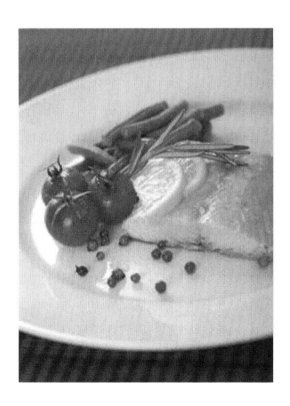

Canned Tuna Salad - 106 kcal

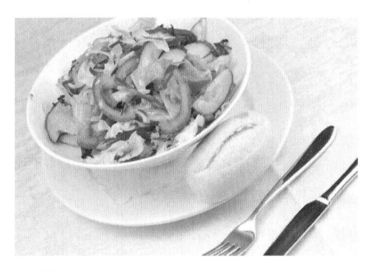

When we first started the 5:2 diet we had this for lunch every fasting day. It is very tasty and filling and we still have it often because it is so simple to do. We sometimes substitute the tuna for a 2 egg omelette which we leave to go cold and chop it up.

106 calories per serving
Preparation - 5 minutes

Ingredients

- 1 tomato
- 2 sticks celery
- 5 thick slices of cucumber,
- 1 spring onion
- ½ tin of tuna in spring water drained

- 1 tbsp of low-fat salad cream
- drizzle of balsamic glaze

Method

Chop or slice all salad ingredients to the size and shape you prefer. Mix the salad cream into the Tuna and stir into the prepared salad. (You can keep the other half in the fridge and use for your next fasting day lunch or use it for a sandwich on a non fasting day.) You can also use mayonnaise if preferred but you will need to add another 50 calories.

Drizzle over a little balsamic glaze and a few basil leaves if you have them for a bit more flavour.

Mussels & Vegetable Sauce - 200 kcal

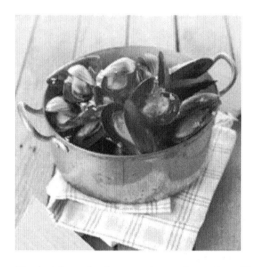

New Zealand cooked mussels are large but if you can't find them, use other fresh mussels instead and steam them just the same. See below for preparation of live mussels. This dish makes a delicious and low calorie starter or for a non fasting day you can add some crusty bread for a more substantial supper.

200 calories per serving
Preparation - 10 minutes
Cooking - 30 minutes

Ingredients

- 1 cal oil spray
- ½ small onion
- 1 clove garlic

- ½ small red pepper
- Sprig of rosemary
- 1 bay leaf
- 40ml / 1½ fl oz / ¼ cup white wine
- 1 small courgette or zucchini
- 200g / 7oz can of chopped tomatoes
- 2 tsp tomato puree
- 25g / 1oz pitted black olives
- 175g / 6oz New Zealand cooked mussels in their shells
- little zest of an orange

Method

Finely chop the onion. Garlic and pepper and gently cook for 4 minutes in the 15 pumps of the oil spray until softened. Add the rosemary and bay leaves with the tomatoes, half of the white wine and then season and bring to the boil. Add the courgette, tomato puree and olives and simmer gently for 10 minutes.

***While this is simmering place the muscles in a streamer and cook over a pan of boiling water covered with a lid. Cook until the mussels all open; throw any away that do not open as they will be bad.

Remove from heat and arrange in a warmed bowl. Take out the rosemary and bay leaves and spoon sauce over the mussels.

****NOTE:

If you are using live mussels, soak them in a bowl of lightly salted water for an hour. Rinse under cold running water and remove any sand by rubbing them lightly with a soft brush. Using a sharp knife remove any 'beards' from the shells. Throw out any broken shells or any opened ones that don't close if tapped firmly with a knife handle. These are dead and must not be eaten as they can cause food poisoning. Rinse the mussels again, drain and put to one side in a colander and use at *** stage.

Notes

Prawn & Fennel Soup - 140 kcal

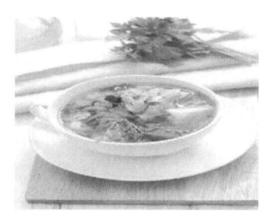

This is a delicious soup that can be served hot or cold.

140 calories per serving

Preparation - 15 minutes

Cooking - 40 minutes

Ingredients

- 1 cal oil spray
- ½ small onion
- 1 medium fennel bulb
- 1 small potato
- 225ml / 8 fl oz or 1 cup water
- 100ml / 4 fl oz / or ½ cup tomato juice or passata
- 40g / 1½ oz cooked small peeled prawns
- 1small tomato
- fresh dill

To serve

- 2 Melba toasts

Method

Halve and slice the onion and fennel bulb. Peel and dice the potato. Skin, de-seed and chop the tomato.

Sauté the onion and fennel in the 5 pumps of the oil for about 4 minutes. Add the potato, water and tomato juice, season with salt. Bring to a simmer and cook on a low heat for about 20-25 minutes, stirring occasionally until the vegetables are cooked.

Let the soup cool slightly and remove the vegetables with a slotted spoon and puree using a food blender or mash with a fork or potato masher until smooth.

Return the puree to the remaining liquid, add the prawns and heat very gently for a few minutes until the soup is heated through.

Snip the dill and stir in the chopped tomato, season to taste and serve with the Melba toasts.

Tuna & White Bean Salad - 160 kcal

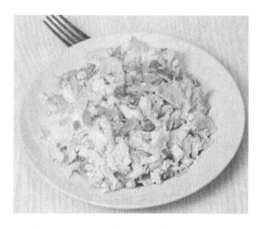

This makes a tasty substantial lunch or will accompany any meat or fish portion

160 calories per serving
Preparation - 10 minutes
Cooking - 5 minutes

Ingredients

- 100g / 3½ oz of cannellini or other white bean

- 1 clove garlic, chopped
- ½ tsp olive oil
- 2 sun-dried tomatoes in oil
- ½ small onion
- ½ of a 185g / 7oz tin of tuna in spring water
- 1 tbsp balsamic vinegar
- Juice of ½ lemon

Method

Heat the olive oil and sauté the garlic for about 30 seconds. Add the drained and rinsed white beans and about half of the lemon juice and warm over a very gentle heat for about 2-3 minutes.

Meanwhile, blot the sun-dried tomatoes of excess oil using kitchen paper and cut into thin strips. Peel and finely chop the onion and add to a bowl with the tomatoes and the partly drained flaked tuna.

Remove the beans from the heat and add them to the bowl. Mix everything together and then add the balsamic vinegar and the rest of the lemon juice, stir and allow the mixture to cool before serving the salad on a large bed of your favourite lettuce leaves.

*** Canned beans are fine but if using dried, cook as directed on packet, drain and rinse as usual.

Cabbage & Prawns - 210 kcal

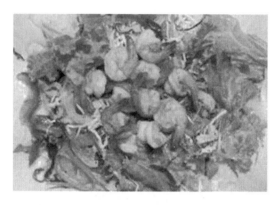

This dish is so quick and easy and I had almost forgotten about it and it is a very low calorie meal. We used to have this a lot when the cabbage was in season and had a good sized solid heart. Very economical and the prawns lift it out of the ordinary.

210 calories per serving
Preparation – 5 minutes
Cooking – 15-20 minutes

Ingredients

- 200g / 7oz sweetheart cabbage or other greens
- 75g fresh or cooked jumbo king prawns
- 1 small onion
- ½ red bell pepper
- 1 cal oil spray
- splash of balsamic vinegar or soy sauce

Method

Remove the outer leaves of the cabbage and cut in half lengthways. Remove the hard core from the centre of the cabbage and then slice it from the tip to the stalk end, discarding any chunky stalk bits. . Wash the cabbage in a bowl of cold water and drain.

Halve and slice the onion and slice the red bell pepper. In a wok or large deep sided frying pan heat 10 pumps of the oil spray and fry the onion for about 3 minutes on a medium heat until starting to soften. Add the red pepper and fry for a further 3-5 minutes then add the cabbage and stir well to bring the onions and pepper from the base of the pan. Add the balsamic or soy sauce, plenty of salt and pepper and then cover the pan and continue to cook for about 5 minutes stirring occasionally.

Check the cabbage is not burning, there should be enough liquid from the cabbage by this time. Carry on cooking on a medium heat, until the cabbage stalks are softened. When cabbage is cooked to your liking, add the prawns. If using raw prawns, continue cooking the dish until they have turned pink and are cooked inside. If using cooked prawns, only heat them through for a couple of minutes at most. Serve on warmed plates with another dash of balsamic on top.

Notes

MEAT & POULTRY

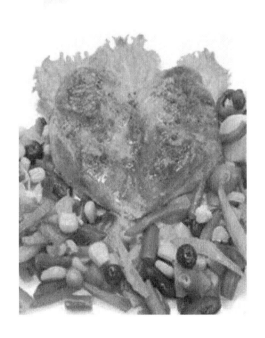

Chicken, Tarragon & Lemon - 175 kcal

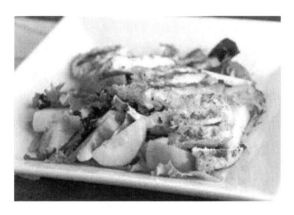

Chicken cooked in tarragon and lemon is a match made in heaven. Just have a crisp green salad in place of the steamed vegetables if preferred.

175 calories per serving
Preparation - 10 minutes
Cooking - 30 minutes

Ingredients

- Juice and zest of ½ lemon
- Small handful of tarragon, stalks removed.
- 1 cal oil spray
- 125g / 4½ oz skinless chicken breast
- 60ml / 2 fl oz / ¼ cup of chicken stock

Method

Preheat the oven to 200°C/gas mark 6. Mix the lemon juice, tarragon leaves and 15 pumps of the oil spray together in a bowl and roll the chicken breast in it. Put in a small oven-proof dish, add the stock around the base of the chicken breast, being careful not to wash off the coating mixture. Pour over any remaining lemon juice and tarragon mixture.

Cover the dish with foil and bake the chicken for 15 minutes. Remove the foil and cook for another 15 minutes, or until the chicken is done. Slice the chicken and serve with a generous helping of steamed broccoli and courgettes as they have very few calories or you can have a crisp green salad.

Curry Coated Chicken - 185 kcal

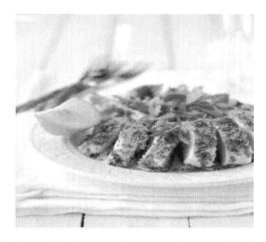

This is a dish that can be eaten hot or cold. Serve with a ratatouille or steamed vegetables or cold with a green salad and the relish

185 calories per serving
Preparation - 15 minutes
Cooking - 30-35 minutes

Ingredients

- 1 chicken breast, boneless and skinless
- 1 garlic clove
- 1 thumbnail size piece of fresh ginger
- ½ green chilli
- 1½ tbsp low-fat natural yoghurt
- ½ tsp ground turmeric
- ½ tsp garam masala

- 1 tsp lime juice
- 1 tsp tomato paste
- wedges of lime or lemon

Relish

- 1 medium tomato
- ¼ of small cucumber
- ½ small red onion
- 1 tbsp chopped flat leafed parsley (optional)

Method

Preheat the oven to 190c / 375F / Gas 5

Crush the garlic clove, peel and finely chop the fresh ginger, deseed and finely chop the green chilli. Mix them together in a bowl with the yogurt, tomato paste, spices, lime juice and seasoning.

Place the chicken breasts on a baking tray and brush them with the paste until covered all over. Bake for 30-35 minutes until the chicken is cooked through.

Make the relish as the chicken is cooking. Finely chop the tomatoes, onion and cucumber and combine with the parsley. Season and chill until needed.

When the chicken is cooked, remove and drain on kitchen paper and serve hot with the relish and lime wedges. Or you can allow to cool and serve with a green salad.

Pork & Apple Medallions - 200 kcal

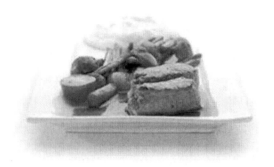

Apple and Pork go together well as the apple is will o
aid digestion. Choose a sweet eating apple to complement
the pork fillet.

200 calories per serving
Preparation – 5 minutes
Cooking – 30-40 minutes

Ingredients

- 2 x 50g / 1¾ oz pork medallions
- ½ tsp oil
- 1 small onion
- ½ tsp sugar
- ½ tsp dried sage
- 75ml / 2½ fl oz / ½ cup chicken stock
- 1 red apple, skinned
- ½ tsp lemon juice

Method

Halve and finely slice the onion.

Fry the onion in the oil in a frying pan for about 5 minutes then add the sugar and cook for another 3-4 minutes until golden. Add the pork and fry 2 minutes each side until browned. Add the sage and stock, bring to a simmer and cook for 20 minutes.

While the pork is cooking, core the apple and cut into quarters and then in half again so you have 8 pieces. Add to the pan and mix in, then cook for another 4-5 minutes until the apples are tender.

Serve with fresh streamed broccoli or a green salad.

Pork & Pine Nuts - 210 kcal

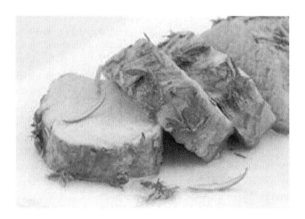

Another quick and simple but impressive dish to cook for the family or for friends and it just creeps into the 200 calorie range.

210 calories per serving
Preparation – 5 minutes
Cooking – 15 minutes

Ingredients

- 125g / 4 oz lean pork fillet
- Small bunch flat leaf parsley
- 1 cal oil spray
- 10g / ½ oz pine nuts
- ½ lemon
- 1 tsp clear honey

Method

Cut the pork fillet into 2cm / ¾ inch thick slices. Lightly coat with the seasoned flour, shaking off any excess.

Heat 10 pumps of oil spray in a large frying pan and cook the pork for 3 minutes each side in a single layer until nicely browned. Remove from the pan and keep warm.

Put another 10 pumps of oil spray into the pan and fry the pine nuts until lightly done. Stir in all of the juice of ½ a lemon and the zest of half of it and stir in the honey as well. Combine to make a sauce.

Return the pork to the pan and scatter with the chopped parsley and cook for a further 3 minutes. Turn the pork during this time so that it is heated through.

Serve with a green salad if fasting or some tagliatelle or other flat pasta for those who are not.

Turkey & Vegetable Loaf - 200 kcal

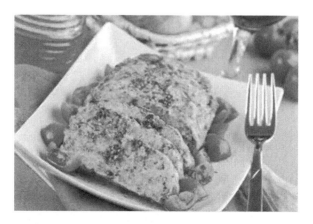

An impressive but easy to make dish. . Alternatively, make a bigger batch and freeze the other portions for a quick and low calorie lunch or serve as a light supper meal for friends. Just cook some baby new potatoes for them and have some broccoli yourself if it is your fasting day

200 calories per serving
***Suitable for freezing
Preparation – 10 minutes
Cooking - 1-1½ hours

Ingredients

- 1 small onion
- 1 garlic clove
- 150g / 5oz minced turkey
- 1 tsp chopped fresh flat leaf parsley
- 1 tsp chopped fresh chives & basil

- 1 egg white
- 1 medium courgette
- 1 medium tomato

Method

Preheat the oven to 190ºC / 375ºF / Gas 5

Finely chop the onion and crush the garlic. Lightly grease a small soufflé dish or loaf tin and line it with baking parchment.

Mix the onion, garlic, herbs and turkey together in a large bowl and season with salt and freshly ground pepper. When well mixed, add the egg white to bind it together. You may want to use your hands to get it mixed well.

Divide the mixture in two and press one portion into the tin, firming it into the corners. Thinly slice the courgette and arrange over the meat. Thinly slice the tomatoes and layer on the courgette. Put the remaining turkey on top of this and press down to firm.

Cover with foil and place in a roasting tin. Pour enough boiling water into the tin to come half way up the meatloaf tin sides. Bake in the oven for 1-1¼ hours removing the foil for the final 20 minutes.

Test the meatloaf is cooked by inserting a knife or skewer into the centre of the loaf. The loaf is cooked if the juices are clear and the loaf has shrunk away from the sides of the tin.

Serve with a good portion of steamed broccoli and courgettes

Vegetable & Meat Soup - 190 kcal

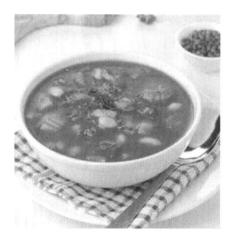

This soup will be very welcome on any type of day. You can use your favourite meat but make sure it is very lean. This recipe is so delicious it won't be around long. If you decide to make a bigger batch it can be kept in the fridge or frozen for another fasting day.

190 calories per serving
***Suitable for freezing
Preparation - 10 minutes
Cooking - 35 minutes

Ingredients

- 15g / ½ oz pearl barley
- 300ml / 10 fl oz / 1¼ beef stock
- 1 tsp dried mixed herbs
- 60g / 2oz lean rump or sirloin steak or lean lamb

or pork fillet
- 1 small carrot
- 25g button mushrooms
- 1 leek
- 1 small onion
- 1 stick or celery
- salt & pepper
- 2 tsp fresh flat leaf parsley – chopped

Method

Cut all the fat from your chosen meat and cut into thin strips.

Dice the carrot, cut the leek in half length ways and wash under cold water to remove any dirt, then cut into 4" pieces and shred length ways. Chop the onion, and then slice the celery.

Add the pearl barley to the stock in a large saucepan with the dried herbs, bring to a simmer and cook for 10 minutes on a low heat with the lid on.

Add the prepared vegetables and the meat to the pan and bring back to the boil, and simmer covered for 15 minutes. Add the mushrooms and cook for a further 5 minutes.

Skim any floating fat or scum from the pan as it cooks and when finished soak up floating fat with kitchen paper.

Serve in deep bowls topped with the parsley

Notes

LESS THAN 300 CALORIES
VEGETARIAN

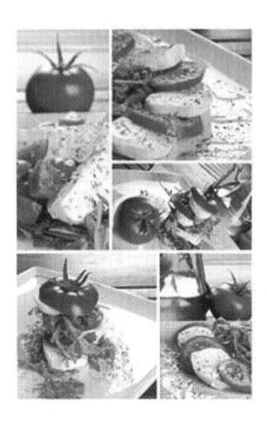

Brown Rice & Tomatoes - 270 kcal

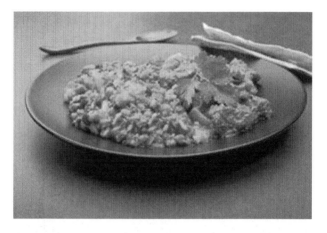

Delicious and healthy because it uses brown rice which is healthier than white rice.

270 calories per serving
Preparation - 5-10 minutes
Cooking - 15 minutes

Ingredients

- ½ tsp crushed red pepper flakes
- 1 clove garlic
- 1 tsp thyme
- 40g / 1½ oz / ¼ cup onions, sliced
- 1 cal oil spray
- 10 cherry tomatoes
- 75g / 3 oz / ½ cup cooked brown rice

Method

Heat 10 pumps of the oil spray in a small pan or skillet and add the finely chopped garlic and sliced onions and cook until golden.

Slice the cherry tomatoes in half and add to the pan with the thyme and crushed red pepper flakes.

Add the cooked brown rice and stir-fry for about 1-2 minutes until heated through and combined.

Serve with a green salad or steamed broccoli

Five Bean Wrap - 295 kcal

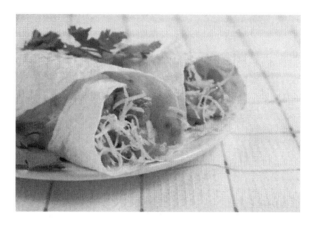

This is a very filling meal and can be eaten for lunch or dinner depending on your schedule. Most food shops now stock many different types of ready cooked beans in either cans or pouches. Try a tin of the mixed bean salad variety which lends itself very well to this recipe.

295 calories per serving
Preparation 5 minutes

Ingredients

- 1 reduced calorie wrap
- 80g / 3oz ready-to-eat mixed beans
- 20g / ¾ oz low calorie or lighter cheddar cheese
- 1 tbsp any salsa
- shredded lettuce

Method

Rinse and drain the beans. Spread your chosen salsa evenly over the whole wrap. Add the drained beans, but leave at least a two inch area free at the bottom of the wrap so that you can fold it over easier.

Put the lettuce on top of the beans and finally grate the cheese evenly over the lettuce. Fold up the bottom of the wrap and roll up the rest.

You may wish to warm the wrap up a bit first as it will be easier to roll but this is not essential.

Hearty Summer Salad - 300 kcal

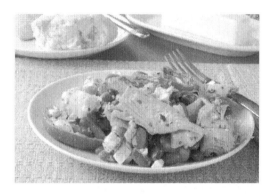

You can get smaller tins of beans if you search or you can use dried beans and cook according to the packet instructions.

300 calories per serving
Preparation - 5-10 minutes

Ingredients
- 100g / 3½ oz. cooked chickpeas
- 100g / 3½ oz. cooked cannellini beans
- 100g / 3½ cooked artichoke hearts
- 1 medium tomato
- ½ small onion
- 2 garlic cloves
- splash olive oil and balsamic vinegar
- a few pinches of dried parsley
- 75g / 2½ oz mixed salad leaves to serve

Method

Drain chickpeas and cannellini beans and put them into a large bowl. Chop artichoke hearts (into eighths if they're whole, or into quarters if they're already halved) and add to bowl. Chop the tomato, dice the onion and crush garlic gloves and add these to the bowl.

Whip olive oil and balsamic vinegar together and pour over the ingredients in the bowl. Add a few generous pinches of dried parsley and salt and pepper to taste.

Stir all the ingredients thoroughly with a large spoon to distribute them evenly and coat them with vinaigrette. Season to taste and serve on a bed of mixed salad.

Mushroom Omelette - 255 kcal

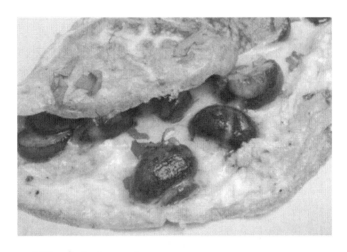

255 calories per serving
Preparation - 5-10 minutes
Cooking - 5-7 minutes

Ingredients

- 75g / 3 oz mushrooms
- 2 medium free range eggs
- Handful of fresh Basil or other preferred herb
- 75g / 3 oz mixed leaf or other salad
- 5 cherry or other small tomatoes
- Dribble of olive oil and balsamic vinegar dressing

Method

Slice or chop the mushrooms and cook in a non stick pan until soft but not shrunk too much, remove from pan and set aside. Wipe out pan and spray with the 1 cal spray oil that you can get from most supermarkets. Lightly beat the eggs together and when pan is hot add the eggs.

Draw the eggs from the side into the middle of the pan until most of the egg liquid has gone from the top of the omelette.

Sprinkle the mushrooms on top evenly, season with salt and freshly ground pepper and when the bottom of the omelette is slightly browned, fold in half, lower heat to minimum and leave to cook very gently for about 1-2 minutes.

Serve with the mixed salad, tomatoes and dressing.

Mushroom Risotto - 290 kcal

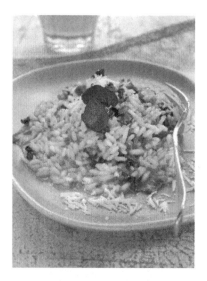

This risotto uses brown rice which is a great source of vitamin B. It is also lower in calories than white rice.

290 calories per serving
***Suitable for freezing
Preparation - 20 minutes
Cooking - 50 minutes

Ingredients

- 5g / ¼ oz dried porcini mushrooms
- 110g / 4 oz mixed mushrooms
- 1 cal oil spray
- 1 small onion
- 1 garlic clove

- 60g / 2 oz brown long grain rice
- 225 ml / 8 fl oz / ½ pint vegetable stock
- 1 tbsp chopped fresh flat leaf parsley

Method

Put the dried porcini mushrooms in a bowl and pour over 75 ml / ¼ cup hot water. Soak for about 20 minutes or until the mushrooms have fully hydrated. Drain but reserve the juice and add it to the stock. Roughly chop the mushrooms.

Finely chop the onion and garlic and using a large pan, sauté in 10 pumps of oil spray for about 5 minutes on a low heat, stirring to avoid burning. Add the rice to the onion mixture and stir well to coat with the oil.

Add the stock, bring to a simmer, lower the heat and cook for 20 minutes or until the liquid has almost gone. Make sure you stir frequently to avoid the risotto sticking to the pan.

Cut the remaining mushrooms into quarters or smaller if using a mixture of larger mushrooms. Add to the rice and stir really well to mix in. Cook for a further 10-15 minutes until all the liquid has been absorbed. Check that the rice has cooked through, adding more hot water or stock if necessary.

Season to taste and add the chopped parsley before serving.

Vegetable & Bean Stew - 270 kcal

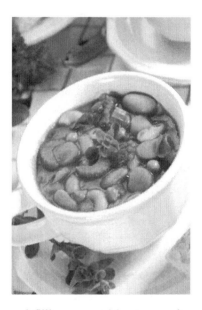

A warm and filling vegetable stew or hearty soup that is very quick to make.

270 calories per serving
Preparation - 10 minutes
Cooking - 20 minutes

Ingredients

- 1 small onion
- 1 stick celery
- 1 medium leek
- 2½ oz frozen peas

- 200g / 7 oz tin cannellini beans or cooked dried beans
- 250ml / 8 fl oz / ½ pint vegetable stock
- 100g / 3½ oz greens (either Spring greens, Sweetheart or Savoy cabbage)

Method

Split the leek in half length ways and wash under running water to remove any soil.

Roughly chop the onion, celery and leek and cook in a couple of sprays of oil until softened. Add the stock and drained beans and cook for about 4 minutes.

Add the greens or cabbage and cook for a further 5-8 minutes. If using Savoy Cabbage, cook until cabbage is as you like it perhaps a further 5-10 minutes according to taste. If you like take out the hard centre stems of the Savoy cabbage and reduce cooking time.

Sprinkle with a little lemon juice and serve.

Notes

FISH

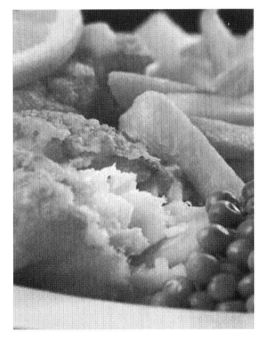

Baked Curried Cod - 260 kcal

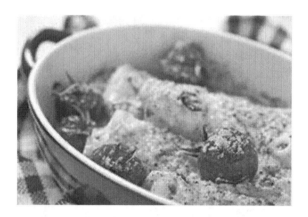

This is a very economical and easy to cook dish and you can also use Monkfish or any other white chunky fish. You could also try it with thick salmon fillets

260 calories per serving
Preparation - 20 minutes
Cooking - 40 minutes

Ingredients

- 1 cal oil spray
- 150g / 5½ oz cod fillet or other firm fish
- 25g / 1 oz fresh white breadcrumbs
- 2 tsp blanched almonds
- 1 tsp Thai green curry paste
- ½ lime
- 50g / 2 oz mixed salad or rocket leaves
- 2 cherry tomatoes

- 1 garlic clove
- dribble olive oil

Method

Pre-heat the oven to 200C or 400F or Gas mark 6

Place the cod fillet in a single layer in a shallow oven-proof dish that has been brushed with the oil spray.

Chop the almonds and mix together with the grated rind of ½ a lime, green curry paste and the breadcrumbs. Stir thoroughly to blend them all in and season with salt and pepper.

Top the fish with the paste, carefully patting onto the top of the fillets so that the fish is well covered. Bake in the pre-heated oven for 35-40 minutes or until the fish is cooked and the top is crusty and brown.

Once the fish is cooking, cut the tomatoes in half and peel and slice the garlic cloves. Push the garlic slivers into the fish 15 minutes before the end of the cooking time, add the tomatoes, spray with oil and bake for the final cooking time.

Serve with the green salad and the juices from the fish and tomato.

Fishcakes & Tomato Sauce - 290 kcal

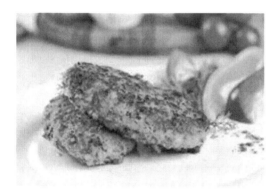

You can make these fishcakes using a combination of any white fish and fresh salmon. The tomato sauce is a welcome change. You should make them ahead of time because they need to be chilled for at least an hour before cooking.

290 calories per serving
***Suitable for freezing
Preparation - 15 minutes plus 1 hour chilling
Cooking - 10-15 minutes

Ingredients

- 110g / 4 oz potatoes
- 110g / 4 oz any white or mixture of fish fillet
- 100ml / 4 fl oz or ½ cup fish stock
- 2 tsp low-fat fromage frais
- 1 tbsp fresh chives
- 20g / ¾ oz dry fresh white or brown

breadcrumbs
- ½ lemon, cut into wedges

Sauce

- 50ml / 2 fl oz / ¼ cup passata or sieved tomatoes
- 1 tbsp low-fat fromage frais
- ½ tsp smoked paprika

Method

Peel and dice the potatoes and cook in boiling water for 10 minutes or until soft. Drain and mash.

Place fish in the stock, bring to the boil and poach on low heat for about 8 minutes. Remove from stock and break into flakes, discarding the skin.

Very carefully, mix together the mashed potato, flaked fish, fromage frais, snipped chives and salt & pepper. Leave the mixture to cool, cover and chill for at least 1 hour.

Divide the mixture into two parts and make each portion into a round patty type fishcake. Coat the fishcakes in the crumbs until covered all over.

Fry in the oil for about 6 minutes each side or until golden and crisp, drain on kitchen paper and keep warm.

Make the sauce by gently heating the passata and when hot but not boiling, remove from heat, stir in the fromage frais and the smoked paprika to taste and serve with the fishcakes and lemon wedges on a bed of baby salad leaves or rocket or try a portion of ratatouille.

Mussels in White Wine - 280 kcal

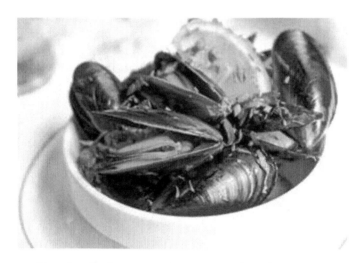

Use the freshest muscles you can find for this dish and it won't disappoint. You really should have some crusty French bread to mop up the juices but if you have this dish on one of your fasting days, that would tip you over your allowance. Save the juice for the next day and have it for lunch with the bread.

Serves 2 – 280 calories per serving
Preparation - 30 minutes
Cooking - 25 minutes

Ingredients

- ½ kg / 1¼ lbs of live mussels
- 1 cal oil spray
- 2-4 large garlic cloves, halved

- 200g / 7 oz tin chopped tomatoes
- 75ml / 2½ fl oz / ½ cup of white wine
- 2 tsp finely chopped fresh leaf parsley
- 1 tsp finely chopped fresh oregano

Method

Soak the live mussels in a bowl of lightly salted water for an hour. Rinse under cold running water and remove any sand by rubbing them lightly with a soft brush. Using a sharp knife remove any 'beards' from the shells.

Throw out any broken shells or any that are open and don't close if tapped firmly with a knife handle. <u>These are dead and must not be eaten as they can cause food poisoning</u>. Rinse the mussels again, drain and put to one side in a colander.

Heat 15 pumps of the oil spray over a low heat in a large pan and sauté the garlic for about a minute but be careful not to burn it and then remove from the pan.

Add the tomatoes and juices, wine and herbs and bring to a simmer. Lower the heat and simmer for about 5 minutes. Tip the mussels into the sauce, cover and simmer for 5-7 minutes, making sure you shake the pan often until all the mussels have opened.

Lift the mussels from the pan with a slotted spoon and discard any unopened ones, spoon into warmed bowls.

Season the sauce to taste and pour over the mussels and top with finely chopped parsley.

Prawn & Chilli Wrap - 240 kcal

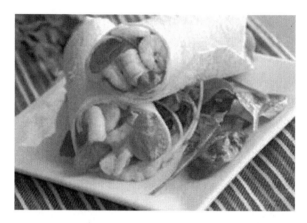

This is a very quick dish to make and the sweet chilli sauce really livens up what could potentially be a bland wrap.

240 calories per serving
Preparation - 2 minutes

Ingredients

- 1 reduced calorie wrap
- 40g / 1½ oz shredded lettuce any kind you like
- 75g / 3 oz cooked prawns
- ½ chopped tomato
- 1 tbsp sweet chilli dipping sauce

Method

Mix the prawns with the chilli sauce. Spread the lettuce over the wrap, making sure you leave a gap clear at the bottom for folding up.

Spread the prawn mixture evenly over the lettuce and then sprinkle the chopped tomato on the top.

Fold up the bottom flap and then roll the remaining wrap gently taking care not to split the folds. It helps if you can warm your wrap in the oven first as it will be more pliable.

Prawn & Dill Soup - 260 kcal

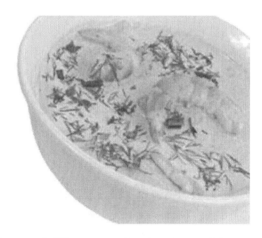

A delicious and filling soup that is substantial enough to be called a stew.

260 calories per serving
Preparation - 5 minutes
Cooking - 10 minutes

Ingredients

- 375ml / ¾ pint / 1½ cups chicken stock
- 1 tbsp fish sauce
- 1 thumb sized piece fresh ginger
- 75g / 2½ oz cooked basmati rice
- juice of ½ lime
- 2 plum tomatoes
- 75g / 2½ oz raw or cooked prawns
- 15g/ ¾ oz chopped dill

Method

Peel and shred the ginger and de-seed and chop the tomatoes.

In a medium pan, bring the stock to a boil and add the fish sauce, shredded ginger, lime juice, chopped tomatoes, dill, prawns and the rice.

Simmer for a few minutes until the prawns are cooked. If using cooked prawns only cook until they are heated through otherwise they will start to shrink and go hard.

Serve in heated bowls with a sprinkling of coriander if liked (optional)

Salmon & Ginger Stir Fry - 295 kcal

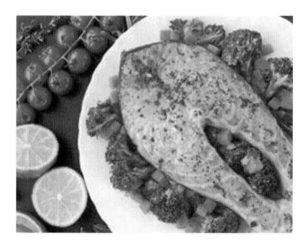

295 calories per serving
Preparation - 10 minutes
Cooking - 10-15 minutes

Ingredients

- 1 x 115g / 4½ oz salmon fillet
- 1 medium head of broccoli
- 1 medium carrot
- 50g / 2 oz mange tout
- ½ inch piece of fresh root ginger
- 1 tbsp light soy sauce
- 1 cal oil spray
- ½ lemon, sliced

Method

Wash the salmon, check for any stray bones and drain on kitchen paper.

Prepare the vegetables by breaking or slicing the broccoli into small florets. Peel the carrot and cut into dice and slice the mange tout into strips, cutting off the top and bottom first. Peel the fresh ginger and again slice into matchstick size strips. Put all the vegetables into a large bowl and stir in 1 tbsp soy sauce, put to one side.

The easiest way to cook the salmon is to bring a shallow pan of water to the boil and when bubbling, slip the salmon fillet into the water, bring back to the boil, put on lid and turn off or remove from the heat. Leave to sit in the hot water without lifting lid for at least 10 minutes. Drain and serve.

In the meantime, heat the 10 pumps of the oil spray in a wok or large frying pan and stir fry the vegetables for about 5 minutes on medium heat until cooked through or to taste. When vegetables are cooked divide between 2 warmed plates and serve the fish on top with a lemon slice and a dash of soy sauce.

Tuna Curry Broth - 260 kcal

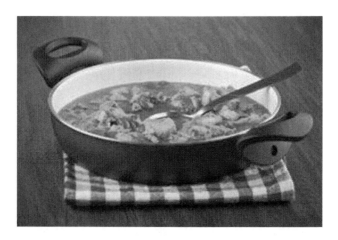

This soup is made using tinned tuna and can be made quickly or in advance and makes a really filling lunch or light dinner.

260 calories per serving
Preparation - 10 minutes
Cooking - 50-60 minutes

Ingredients

- 50g / 2 oz canned tuna in spring water
- 5g / ¼ oz butter
- 1 small onion
- 1 clove garlic
- 2 tsp plain flour
- 1 tsp mild curry powder
- 100g / 3½ oz canned plum tomatoes

- 1 tbsp white rice
- 1 small courgette
- 25ml / 1 fl oz / ⅛ cup single cream

Method

Finely chop the onion and garlic clove and wash and finely dice the courgette. Drain the tuna but reserve the water and make up to 600ml or 2½ cups with boiling water.

Melt the butter in a large pan and sauté the onion and garlic for 5minutes or until softened. Stir in the flour and curry powder, and cook off for 2 minutes, stirring constantly. Add the water mixture a little at a time stirring well and bring to a low simmer. Add the tomatoes, breaking up with the spoon, return to the boil, add the rice, cover and simmer gently for about 10 minutes.

Finally, add the tuna and courgette and cook for a further 15 minutes or until the courgette and rice are cooked. Stir in the cream and adjust the seasoning to taste. Simmer for another 2-3 minutes to heat thoroughly and serve in warmed bowls.

Tuna Fishcakes - 275 kcal

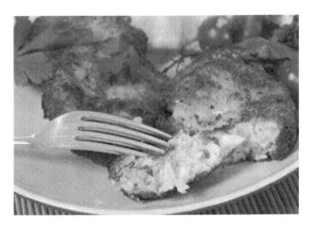

Tasty tuna fishcakes that are so full of protein and low in calories too.

275 calories per serving
Preparation - 10 minutes
Cooking 10 - 15 minutes

Ingredients

- 1 large egg
- ¼ tsp ground cumin powder
- 1 tbsp finely chopped onion
- 1 7oz can tuna fish in water

Method

Spray frying pan or skillet with 1 cal cooking spray or the oil & water mix and heat on medium.

Mix all ingredients together well and divide into manageable sizes perhaps 4 or 6 as the smaller they are, the quicker they will cook and the easier they will be to handle.

When pan is hot, cook on both sides until they are a light brown colour, feel and look firm and there is no liquid or egg flowing out of them.

Enjoy with a green salad or good portion of steamed broccoli.

Tuna Steaks & Beans - 270 kcal

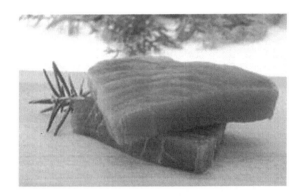

This recipe is still one of our favourites because you can change the Tuna to almost any other meat or fish. Try is with fishcakes, salmon fillets, steak etc, the variations are endless.

270 calories per serving
Preparation - 5 minutes
Cooking - 10 minutes

Ingredients

- 1 x 100g / 4 oz Tuna Steaks
- 75g / 2½ oz mixed salad leaves or rocket
- 200g / 7 oz cannellini beans, drained & rinsed
- 2 garlic cloves, sliced
- 4 spring onions, sliced
- ½ tsp olive oil
- 1 tbsp lemon juice

Method

Cook Tuna for a few minutes each side until cooked as you like it, or if using frozen cook according to packet instructions.

I find a good way to cook the tuna steak is to bring a shallow pan of water to the boil and when bubbling, slip the fish into the water, bring back to the boil, put on lid and turn off or remove from heat. Leave to sit in the hot water without lifting lid for at least 12 minutes. Drain and serve.

At the same time, in a small pan, sauté the garlic in the olive oil for a few seconds taking care not to burn it and then add the drained and rinsed beans and lemon juice. Cook for a few more minutes and spoon over the arranged salad leaves. Sprinkle over the spring onions, drizzle some balsamic glaze and serve with the Tuna steaks.

Notes

MEAT & POULTRY

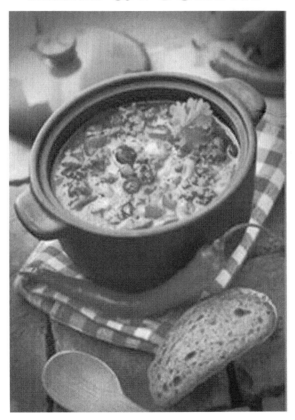

Beef Strips with Pak Choy
- 270 kcal

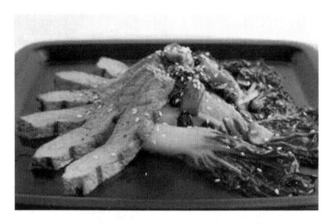

Pak Choy is used a lot in oriental cooking with good reason. It is low in calories and goes well with almost anything.

270 calories per serving
Preparation – 10 minutes
Cooking – 10 minutes

Ingredients

- 1 cal oil spray
- 1 small to medium sirloin steak
- Small piece fresh ginger
- 1 garlic clove
- 2 spring onions
- 2 tsp soy sauce

- 1 pak choy
- 25g / 1 oz mange tout or snow peas

Method

Trim all the fat off the steak and cut it into very thin slices. Peel and grate the ginger. Slice the spring onions. Crush the garlic. Cut the pak choy lengthways into quarters.

Heat 5 pumps of the oil spray in a wok and brown the beef. When browned, add the ginger and onions and stir fry for 2 minutes. Add the soy sauce and keep warm.

Steam the pak choy and mange tout until tender, serve with the beef.

Beef with Green Lentils - 240 kcal

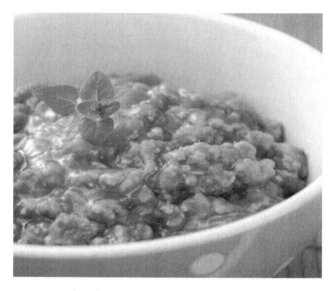

This is a variation on spaghetti bolognese that freezes really well if you want to make bigger batches. You can have this as a topping for a jacket potato, but do not eat the skin or your calories will rocket. Also have it with some steamed broccoli and courgettes which are very few calories.

240 calories per serving
***Suitable for freezing
Preparation – 5 minutes
Cooking – 40-45 minutes

Ingredients

- 65g / 2½ oz lean minced beef
- 1 small onion
- ½ tsp mustard
- 2 tsp Worcestershire sauce
- 2 tsp tomato puree
- 100g / 3½ oz canned chopped tomatoes
- 35g / 1 oz green lentils

Method

Peel and chop the onion and rinse the lentils in cold water, drain. Cook the mince and onion in a non-stick pan on a medium heat until the meat is brown all over, stirring often.

Add the mustard, some freshly ground black pepper and salt to taste. Next add the Worcestershire sauce, chopped tomatoes plus one can of water and finally the tomato puree.

Stir to combine all the ingredients and bring to a low simmer. Stir in the rinsed lentils and cover and simmer for 30 minutes until sauce is nicely thickened.

Add some chopped chives if wished (optional) and serve with some streamed vegetables or a 200g / 7 oz jacket potato (add 154 calories) but don't eat the skin (or add another 118 calories).

Chicken & Apricot - 260 kcal

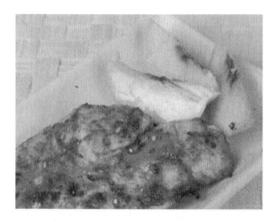

Chicken and apricots go well together and make a nice change from the usual stuffing's for chicken.

260 calories per serving
Preparation – 10 minutes
Cooking – 25 minutes

Ingredients

- 1 skinless boneless chicken breast
- 1 small onion
- 1 garlic clove
- 1 cal oil spray
- 2 dried apricots
- 50g / 2 oz spinach
- 2 tsp cumin
- 2 tsp clear honey

Method

Halve and thinly slice the onion and garlic. Finely chop the apricots and chop the spinach.

Heat the oven to 200°C / fan 180°C / gas 6

Sauté the onion and garlic in a frying pan with 10 pumps of the oil spray for 5 minutes. Season well and add the apricots, spinach and 1 tsp cumin and cook for a further minute or two.

Make a cut in the chicken across the side to form a pocket and stuff the cooked mixture into the breast. Rub the remaining cumin into the top of the chicken and season. Pour over the honey, put in a small dish and bake for 20 minutes until cooked.

Serve with a portion of green beans or steamed broccoli.

Chicken & Avocado Bake - 290 kcal

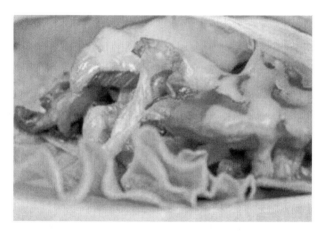

This is a typically French dish which is very easy to cook. The fat content comes mostly from the avocado but it consists of mostly heart-healthy mono-unsaturated fats.

290 calories per serving
Preparation - 5 minutes
Cooking - 20 minutes

Ingredients

- 4 oz / 120g boneless chicken breast
- 1 cal oil spray
- 1 oz extra lean ham or prosciutto
- 1 slice avocado
- 2 slices fresh tomato
- 1 oz low fat hard cheese

Method

Preheat oven to 230C / 210 fan / 450F (very hot).

Pat dry the chicken and remove any visible fat. Place chicken between 2 sheets of cling film or other suitable bag and flatten to a ½ - ¾ inch steak. Lightly season to taste.

Add 10 pumps of the oil spray to a hot sauté pan and fry the chicken until browned on both sides. Remove from the pan and place into a small oven-proof dish.

Fry the ham very quickly in the hot pan juices until just starting to turn brown.

Place ham on top of the chicken, then the tomato, avocado and cheese. Bake until cheese starts to bubble. Remove from oven and serve with a green salad or a big portion of steamed broccoli.

Chicken & Tomatoes - 270 kcal

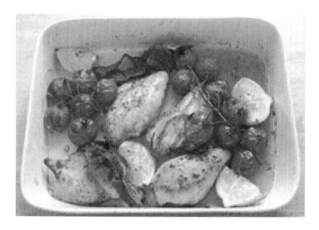

A very quick lunch or dinner meal that is easy to cook and delicious to eat.

270 calories per serving
Preparation - 5 minutes
Cooking - 15 minutes

Ingredients

- 1skinless boneless chicken breast
- 2 tsp seasoned flour
- 1 cal oil spray
- 1 small onion
- 2 stick celery
- 50g / 2 oz cherry or baby plum tomatoes
- ½ lemon

- 2 tsp white wine vinegar
- 1 tbsp chopped basil leaves
- Rocket or baby salad leaves to serve.

Method

Halve and slice the onion, thinly slice the celery and halve the tomatoes.

Cut the chicken breasts in half to form 2 thin breasts. Place between 2 sheets of cling film and flatten a bit more using a suitable heavy object to form thin escallops without destroying the flesh.

Place the seasoned flour on a plate and dip the chicken breast in it to evenly coat, shake off any excess.

Heat 10 pumps of the oil spray over a medium heat in a non stick frying pan and fry the chicken pieces until they are brown on both sides and cooked through.

Remove from the pan and add the celery and onion and fry for 4 minutes.

Next put in the tomatoes and cook for a further 4 minutes until starting to soften. Add the vinegar and the chicken again and cook through for 3-4 minutes and then stir in the chopped basil. Serve with salad leaves of choice.

Chicken & Mixed Vegetables - 280 kcal

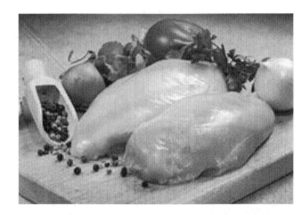

This is a very easy dish to prepare and cook. The chicken breast stays lovely and moist and the vegetables cook just perfectly. As a bonus there will be very little washing up and even if you leave it longer in the oven, the flavours will just increase.

280 calories per serving
Preparation - 10 minutes
Cooking - 50-60 minutes

Ingredients

- 1 x chicken breast approx 125g / 4½ oz
- ½ medium onion sliced
- 1 small courgette or zucchini sliced
- 100g / 4 oz green beans cut into half
- 1 medium tomato sliced
- 75g / 3 oz broccoli florets

- 1 chicken stock cube

Method

Make a parcel using foil or small roasting bag and place the vegetables in the foil or bag. Lay the chicken breast on top of the vegetables. Make up the stock cube as directed and pour some into the chicken parcel, not too much, just enough to keep the parcels moist.

Season well with salt and pepper. Add a tsp of your favourite dried herbs or a handful of fresh if you have them. Fold up and seal the parcel, not too tightly or the heat won't penetrate and the vegetables won't cook through. Place in an oven proof dish and cook for a minimum of 50-60 minutes at 190c.

Chicken, & Pesto Broth - 320 kcal

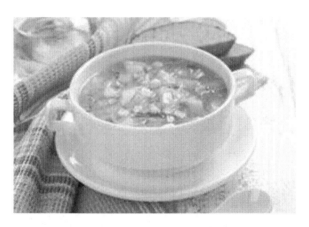

This is a delicious, nutritious and filling broth that you can freeze and save for another fasting day if you do bigger batches or have it for lunch with some crusty bread on a normal day.

320 calories per serving
***Suitable for freezing
Preparation - 10 minutes
Cooking - 20 - 25 minutes

Ingredients

- 250 ml / 8 fl oz / 1 cup of chicken stock
- 1 small skinless chicken breast
- 1 carrot
- 25g / 1oz Orzo pasta
- ¼ Savoy cabbage

- 1 spring onions
- 2 tsp pesto

Method

Peel the carrots and cut into lengths. Core the cabbage and slice roughly. Top and tail the spring onions and slice.

In a large pan, place the stock, whole chicken breast and carrots, bring to a simmer and cook on a low heat for 5 minutes.

Add the pasta, cabbage, spring onions and salt and pepper. Simmer for a further 5 minutes until the pasta is tender and the chicken is cooked through.

Using a ladle, remove the chicken from the pan and slice. Portion out the broth using a ladle into however many portions you are serving. Top with the sliced chicken and ½ tbsp of pesto per serving.

Chicken, Pea & Rice Soup- 320 kcal

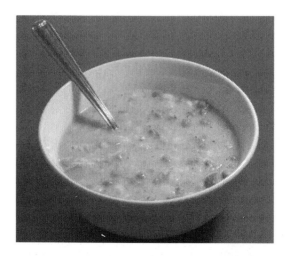

I know this is called a soup but the rice makes is a filling lunch or dinner meal. Try it as you should have the majority of the ingredients to hand and can even use any leftover chicken.

320 calories per serving
***Suitable for freezing
Preparation – 5 minutes
Cooking – 10-15 minutes

Ingredients
- 375ml / ¾ pt / 1¾ cups chicken stock
- 25g / 1 oz long grain rice
- 1 small cooked chicken breast or leftover chicken
- 25g / 1 oz defrosted frozen peas

- small handful basil leaves

Method

Heat the chicken stock in a medium pan, add the rice and cook for 8-10 minutes. Add the shredded chicken breast and peas and cook for a further 2 minutes. Season and add the torn basil leaves and serve.

Chicken & Pepper Couscous - 350 kcal

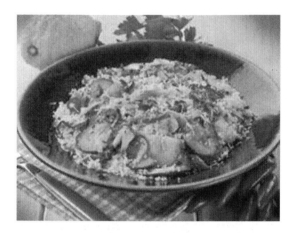

This is a handy salad dish to make because you can use the ready cooked roasted chicken breasts or leftover chicken.

350 calories per serving
Preparation – 10 minutes
Cooking – 10 minutes

Ingredients

- 50g / 2 oz dried couscous
- ½ red bell pepper
- 1 spring onion/scallion
- 25g / 1 oz raisins
- 1 red chilli
- 1 small courgette/zucchini
- juice of ½ lemon

- 1 small roasted chicken breast
- handful salad leaves

Method

De-seed and cut the pepper into small chunks. Slice the spring onions and the chilli, seeds removed if preferred. Cut the courgette into thin ribbons using a vegetable peeler.

Mix the couscous, onions, pepper chunks, chilli and raisins into a large bowl. Heat up the chicken stock and pour over the couscous mixture. Cover and let stand for 10 minutes.

Fluff up with a fork and then stir lemon juice. Season well and serve with the sliced chicken breast and salad leaves.

Lamb & Apricot Casserole - 290 kcal

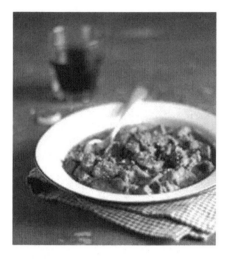

This is a fruity meat casserole with a bit of a kick. The lamb and apricots complement each other and the spices perk it all up.

290 calories per serving
***Suitable for freezing
Preparation – 10 minutes
Cooking – 1 hour 20 minutes

Ingredients

- 110g / 4oz lean lamb
- ½ tsp ground cinnamon
- ½ tsp ground coriander
- ½ tsp ground cumin
- ½ tsp olive oil

- 1 small red onion
- 1 garlic clove
- 100g / 3½ oz chopped canned tomatoes
- 2 tsp tomato puree
- 30g / 1 oz ready to eat dried apricots
- 1 tsp sugar
- 75ml / 2½ fl oz / ¼ cups vegetable stock

Method

Pre-heat the oven to 180°C/350°F/Gas 4

Trim all fat from the meat and cut into 2.5cm/1 inch chunks. Finely chop the red onion and crush the garlic.

Put the meat into a bowl and mix in the spices and the oil. Make sure all of the pieces are coated well.

Heat a non-stick pan until it is hot and then add the lamb. Reduce the heat and cook stirring for 5 minutes until browned all over. Remove the lamb from the pan using a slotted spoon and put into a large ovenproof casserole.

Now cook the onions, garlic, tomatoes and puree for 5 minutes in the same pan, stirring in any juices left from the meat. Season to taste and add the whole apricots and sugar and then the stock and bring to the boil.

Remove from heat and spoon the mixture over the lamb in the casserole, cover and cook for 1 hour. Remove the lid and cook for another 10 minutes

Serve with steamed broccoli on a fasting day and rice or couscous on a normal day.

Lamb & Lentil Curry
- 280 kcal

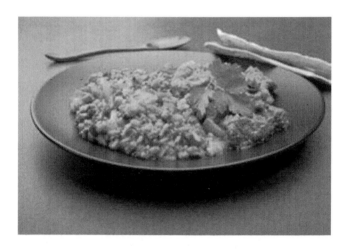

A warm and filling curry that can be served with a low calorie poppadom for added satisfaction.

280 calories per serving
***Suitable for freezing
Preparation - 10 minutes
Cooking - 30 minutes

Ingredients

- 1 medium onion
- 80g / 3 oz lean minced lamb
- 1 garlic clove
- 1 tbsp balti curry paste
- 150 ml / 5 fl oz low salt beef stock

- 2 tbsp canned chopped tomatoes
- 90g / 3 oz baby spinach leaves
- 3 tbsp drained canned green lentils

Method

Slice the onion, crush the garlic and wash the baby spinach.

In a large heavy based saucepan fry the onion in a couple of sprays of 1 cal oil spray or oil and water mix for about 3 minutes, stirring often. Put in the minced lamb and cook for a further 2 minutes until nicely browned.

Add the garlic and cook for another minute. Add the balti paste, stock and tomatoes and cook over a low heat for 15 minutes, stirring often to avoid sticking.

Finally add the spinach and lentils and cook for a further 5 minutes. Serve with a handful of chopped coriander if liked (optional).

Lamb's Liver & Apple - 285 kcal

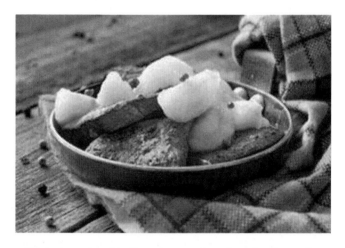

Delicious lamb's liver is very low in calories and very healthy.

285 calories per serving
Preparation - 10 minutes
Cooking - 25 minutes

Ingredients

- 200g / 7 oz swede
- 100g / 3½ oz lamb's liver
- 2 spring onions/scallions
- 1 tbsp milk
- 1 cal oil spray
- 1 small apple

- 75ml / 2½ fl oz unsweetened apple juice
- 2 tsp balsamic vinegar
- ½ tsp dried tarragon

Method

Peel and dice the swede, chop the spring onions, slice the lambs liver into thin strips and core and cut the apple into 8 wedges.

Cook the swede in a pan of boiling water for about 10 minutes, drain. Add the chopped spring onions and milk and stir. Place a lid on and keep warm.

In a non-stick pan or wok, stir fry the liver in 10 pumps of the oil spray for 1 minute then add the apple wedges and stir fry for a further minute. Add the apple juice, balsamic vinegar and tarragon and cook on high for 3-5 minutes until liquid has almost gone.

Mash the swede and season to taste. Serve liver on a bed of mashed swede with any pan juices poured over.

Pork Chilli & Beans - 300 kcal

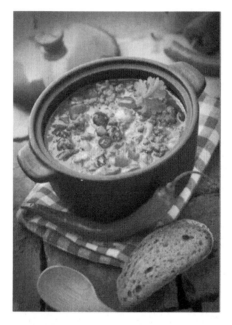

A one pot dish that you will eat over and over again, it's that good. Use tenderloin of pork a really tender cut of pork and good value as there's no waste.

300 calories per serving
Preparation - 10 minutes
Cooking - 30 - 35 minutes

Ingredients

- 1 cal oil spray
- 100g / 3½ oz pork tenderloin
- 1 small onion

- 1 garlic clove
- pinch chilli flakes or crushed chilli
- ½ tsp cumin
- ½ red bell pepper
- 100g / 3½ oz canned chopped tomatoes
- 100ml / 3½ fl oz / ½ cup chicken stock
- 60g / 2½ oz small salad potatoes
- 25g / 1 oz green beans

Method

Dice the pork into bite sized pieces. Halve and slice the onion and then peel and slice the garlic. De-seed the red pepper and cut into chunks. Wash and halve the salad potatoes.

Top and tail the green beans and cut in half.

Heat 5 pumps of the oil spray in a large pan and season and brown the pork. When browned all over, remove from pan and add the onion and garlic and sauté for a minute.

Add the chilli, cumin and pepper and cook for a further 2 minutes. Put the pork back in the pan with the tomatoes and stock and bring to a simmer. Add the potatoes and cook for about 10-15 minutes, stirring occasionally until the potatoes and meat are tender.

Add the green beans and cook for a further 5 minutes. Season and serve.

Pork & Mixed Peppers - 300 kcal

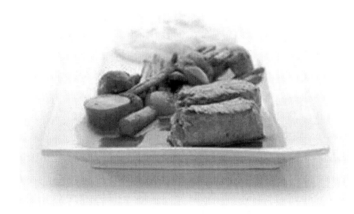

Very quick and easy supper dish that can easily be served to guests with extra vegetables or new potatoes

300 calories per serving
Preparation - 10 minutes
Cooking - 30 minutes

Ingredients

- 1 cal oil spray
- 1 small onion
- 1 cloves garlic
- ½ red pepper
- ½ yellow pepper
- 100g / 3½ oz canned chopped tomatoes
- 1 pork escallop

- 2 tsp red wine vinegar
- 1 tsp olive oil

Method

Finely chop the onion and de-seed and finely slice the peppers, finely slice the garlic clove. Trim the fat from the meat.

In a large frying pan, heat 10 pumps of the oil spray and cook the onions for 5 minutes until soft. Add the sliced garlic and cook for a further minute. Add the peppers and 2 tbsp water and cover and cook for 10 minutes. Add the tomatoes and cook for 10-15 minutes uncovered until the peppers are soft.

Brush the pork with a few pumps of the oil spray and grill or griddle for 3-5 minutes each side depending on taste. Leave to rest covered with foil.

Mix the 1 tsp olive oil and the vinegar with the crushed garlic. Make a bed of the pepper mixture on a warmed plate, top with the pork and drizzle over the dressing.

Serve with steamed broccoli if fasting or potatoes and vegetables if not.

Pork & Roasted Vegetables - 265 kcal

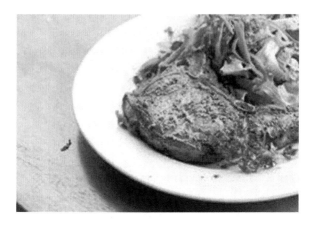

Simple dish to prepare and cook but filling nevertheless.

265 calories per serving
Preparation – 10 minutes
Cooking – 25-30 minutes

Ingredients

- 1 medium carrot
- ½ red pepper
- 1 small courgette
- 1 cal oil spray
- 1 good size pork chop
- ¼ tsp paprika
- 50g / 2 oz watercress

Method

Preheat the oven to 200°C / fan 180°C / Gas 6

Peel and slice the carrot and slice the courgette. Deseed and chop the red pepper. Place in a roasting tin and spray with the oil spray. Season and roast for 25-30 minutes.

Meantime, heat a grill or griddle pan. Sprinkle the pork chops with the paprika and cook for 5 minutes each side.

Remove the vegetables from the oven and stir in the watercress. Serve with the pork chop.

Spicy Chicken Pitta - 275 kcal

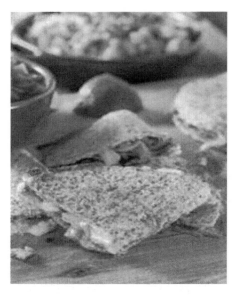

275 calories per serving
Preparation - 5 minutes
Marinating - 30 minutes
Cooking: 10minutes

Ingredients

- 2 spring onions, chopped finely
- 2 garlic cloves, chopped finely
- juice ½ lemon
- 1 tsp honey
- ½ tsp paprika
- ¼ tsp mild chilli powder
- ½ chicken breast fillet

- 1 pita bread
- small amount iceberg lettuce

Method

Finely chop the spring onion and garlic and mix together with the lemon juice, honey, paprika and chilli powder to form a marinade.

Cut the chicken breast into small lumps about 2.5cm or 1 inch square. Mix the chicken with the marinade and leave it in the fridge for at least 30 minutes, longer if possible.

Pre-heat your grill to the highest setting and when ready, grill the chicken for roughly 8 minutes, turning over half way through. The chicken pieces will be ready when nicely crisp and brown.

Remove from grill and quickly toast your pita bread. Make a pocket in the pita and fill with the shredded lettuce and cooked chicken

Notes

LESS THAN 400 CALORIES VEGETARIAN

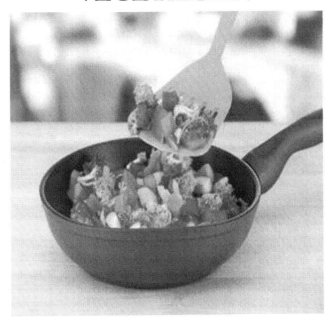

Butternut Squash Risotto - 365 kcal

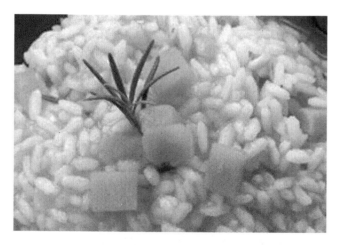

Risotto is a very easy dish to master once you get the hang of it. This recipe freezes well if you want to make a bigger batch so that you can have more ready meals in the freezer.

365 calories per serving
***Suitable for freezing
Preparation – 10 minutes
Cooking – 20-25 minutes

Ingredients

- 1 small onion
- 1 cal oil spray
- 1 x 125g / 4½ oz butternut squash
- 75g / 2½ oz carnnaroli or arborio risotto rice
- 300ml / 10 fl oz / 1¼ cups vegetable stock

- 1 tbsp grated parmesan

Method

Chop the onion finely. Peel and dice the butternut squash or pumpkin.

Heat 10 pumps of oil spray in a large pan and fry the onion until softened. Add the rice and stir until coated in the oil. Add the squash and half the hot stock and stir well. Cook, stirring often until most of the stock has been absorbed. Then add a little stock at a time, again stirring until absorbed.

Repeat this until all the stock has been used and the rice and squash are cooked. The rice should have a little bite but not grainy. Add more stock or hot water if needed.

Add the cheese to the rice and stir well. Cover the pan and leave to sit for 1 minute.

Season well and dish out into warmed bowls. Add a very tiny splash of olive oil to each bowl and serve.

Golden Rice & Onions - 365 kcal

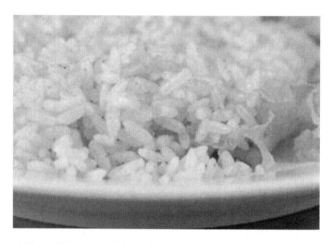

This dish has a hint of Indian spices and the turmeric gives the rice a warming yellow colour. Leave the topping onions out if not to your taste or too much bother to do but they do add a little more colour and flavour.

365 calories per serving
***Suitable for freezing
Preparation - 10 minutes
Cooking - 25-30 minutes

Ingredients

- 45g / 1¾ oz basmati rice
- 15g / ½ oz red lentils
- 1 bay leaf
- 1 cardamom pod, split
- ½ tsp ground turmeric

- 2 cloves
- ½ tsp cumin seeds
- ½ cinnamon stick
- 1 small onion
- 60g / 2 oz cauliflower florets
- 1 small carrot
- 25g / 1 oz frozen peas
- 15g / ½ oz sultanas
- 150ml / 5 fl oz / ¾ cup vegetable stock
- salt & pepper
- 2 tsp chopped fresh coriander (optional)

For the Onions

- ½ tsp vegetable oil
- ½ small red onion
- 1½ small white onion
- ½ tsp caster sugar

Method

Peel and dice the carrot, break the cauliflower into small florets. Put the carrot, cauliflower, onion, rice, lentils, spices, bay leaf, peas and sultanas into a large pan. Season and thoroughly mix.

Pour over the stock, bring to the boil, cover and simmer for 15 minutes stirring occasionally to avoid the rice sticking. Add more stock if it runs dry before the rice is cooked.

When the rice is tender, remove, cover and it let stand for about 10 minutes or until all the liquid has been absorbed. Take out the bay leaf, cardamom pods, cloves and cinnamon stick.

While the rice is cooking, shred the onions, heat the oil in a frying pan and fry the onions over a medium heat for 4 minutes until just starting to soften. Add the sugar, turn up the heat and cook, stirring all the time for a further 2-3 minutes until golden but not burnt.

Stir the rice mixture through and serve on warmed plates with the onions on top and sprinkled with the chopped coriander if liked.

Notes

204

Low Fat Pesto Tagliatelle - 350 kcal

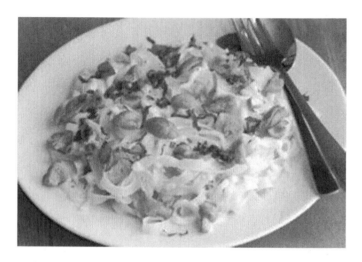

Pesto sauce is quite high in fat content but this sauce uses fromage frais instead of oil and is therefore much healthier. You can also use any colour pasta you choose or try a combination of green and white tagliatelli.

350 calories per serving
Preparation - 10 minutes
Cooking - 15 minutes

Ingredients

- 60g / 2¼ oz chestnut or other mixed mushrooms
- 40ml / 1½ oz / ⅓ cup vegetable stock
- 45g / 1¾ oz asparagus

- 75g / 2½ oz fresh tagliatelle
- 100g / 3½ oz ready to eat artichoke hearts
- Parmesan shavings

Pesto sauce

- 1 garlic clove
- 15g / ½ oz fresh basil leaves
- 1½ tbsp low-fat natural fromage frais
- ½ tbsp grated Parmesan cheese
- salt & pepper

Method

Make the pesto sauce by either using a blender or finely chopping the basil and mixing it well with all the other ingredients.

To make the pasta, slice the mushrooms, place in a small pan with the stock, bring to the boil and poach in the vegetable stock for 4 minutes. Drain and set aside.

Rinse out the pan, trim and cut the asparagus into 5cm (2") lengths and cook in boiling water for 3-4 minutes, drain and also set aside.

Cook the pasta as directed on the packet, drain, sprinkle with a little olive oil to stop it sticking, return to the pan. Add the mushrooms, cooked asparagus, and the drained and halved artichoke hearts and cook on a very low heat for about 2 minutes. Remove from heat and stir in the pesto sauce and serve with a few shredded basil leaves and the parmesan shavings.

Vegetable & Potato Bake - 350 kcal

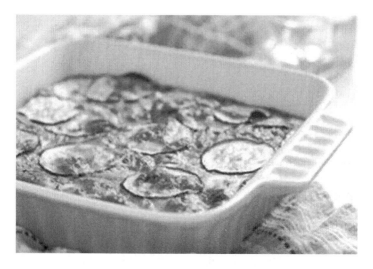

This is a substantial vegetable dish with a potato and cheese topping. This is unusual for a low calorie meal so enjoy it.

350 calories per serving
Preparation – 10 minutes
Cooking – 25-30 minutes

Ingredients

- 1 small onion
- 1 garlic clove
- ½ red pepper and ½ green pepper
- 1 small aubergine
- 1 small courgette (zucchini)
- 1 200g /7oz canned chopped tomatoes

- ½ tbsp dried mixed herbs
- 2 tsp tomato puree
- 225g / 8 oz potatoes
- 25g / 1oz grated low fat cheese

Method

Finely chop the onions and garlic. Deseed and halve and slice the peppers. Top and tail the aubergine and cut into small chunks. Trim and thinly slice the courgettes.

Put the onion, garlic, peppers, dried herbs, tomato puree and the chopped tomatoes in a large pan. Bring to the boil, cover and simmer gently for 10 minutes, stirring occasionally.

Stir in the aubergine and courgettes and cook uncovered for another 10 minutes, giving it the occasional stir.

While the vegetables are cooking, peel and cut the potatoes into 2.5cm / 1 inch pieces. Boil them for 7-10 minutes until cooked through and then drain.

Put the vegetables into a small ovenproof dish. Place the potatoes on top of the vegetable mixture, sprinkle the cheese on top of the potatoes.

Preheat your grill to medium and grill the dish for 5 minutes until the cheese is bubbling and the potatoes are getting golden and crispy. Serve on warmed plates with nothing else.

Mushroom Risotto - 365 kcal

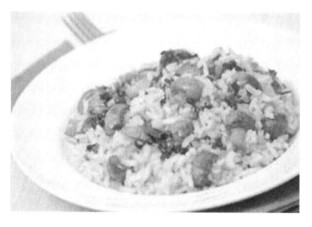

Risotto is a really easy dish to cook once you get into the swing of it. You can use any variety of mushrooms you like.

365 calories per serving
Preparation - 5-10 minutes
Cooking - 20-25 minutes

Ingredients

- 1 small onion
- 125g / 4½ oz mixed mushrooms
- 1 cal oil spray
- 80g / 3 oz risotto rice
- 250ml / 8 fl oz / 1 cup of hot vegetable stock
- 20g / 1 oz Parmesan cheese, grated
- A small handful of flat leaved parsley, chopped

Method

Chop the onions and garlic, and wipe the mushrooms before also chopping them. Warm 10 pumps of the oil spray in a large pan, add the onions and garlic and cook gently for 2 minutes. Then add the mixed mushrooms and cook for another minute or so.

Add the risotto rice and stir well to coat the rice with the juices for about a minute. Add enough of the hot stock to cover the rice and cook, stirring constantly until the liquid has been absorbed.

Add more hot stock a little at a time and allow it to be absorbed also, (for best results you should keep the stock hot in a separate pan on the stove).

Repeat this process, stirring as you do, until the rice is ready, there should be a hint of grain but not too hard. Add more boiling water if necessary when stock has been used up.

Remove from heat, stir in the Parmesan and chopped parsley, check the seasoning and allow to stand for 1 minute before serving on warmed plates.

Pasta & Cherry Tomatoes- 325 kcal

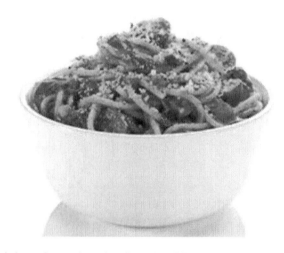

A low fat recipe that is quite filling as well as being tasty and very quick and easy to make

325 calories per serving
Preparation - 5 minutes
Cooking - 15 minutes

Ingredients

- 100g / 4 oz cherry tomatoes
- 3 black olives
- 1 clove of garlic, peeled
- A handful of basil
- 1 cal oil spray
- 75g / 3 oz fresh spaghetti pasta
- bag mixed salad leaves or rocket

Method

Chop the tomatoes, olives and garlic. Put them into a bowl with some basil, then spray with the oil spray until coated well and stir.

Cook the pasta as directed. Once the pasta is cooked, drain and rinse through with boiling water and return to the pan. Add the tomato mixture from the bowl and stir over a very low heat.

Add salt and black pepper, and serve immediately with a big helping of mixed salad leaves.

Penne & Pepper Sauce - 375 kcal

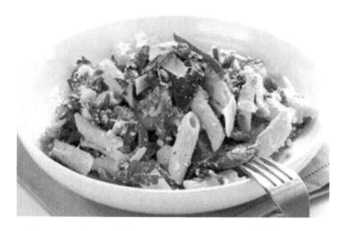

Pasta makes a filling supper dish but don't have it too often with meat. This only uses vegetables so is very healthy.

375 calories per serving
Preparation - 15 minutes
Cooking - 20 minutes

Ingredients

- ½ red and ½ yellow pepper
- 1 small red onion
- 1 cloves of garlic
- 1 cal oil spray
- 85g / 3 oz fresh penne pasta

Method

Remove the seeds and membranes from the peppers. Rub the skins with a little olive oil and place them, skin sides up, on a piece of foil under a hot grill. Once the skins have burnt and turned brown, remove from grill and allow cool slightly. Pull off the skin, slice and put into a small mixing bowl.

Chop the onion and garlic. Cook the pasta as directed on the pack. While the pasta is cooking, put 10 pumps of the oil spray in a large frying pan and gently fry the onion and garlic. Add the peppers and juices from the bowl and continue cooking, stirring them together. Add some pasta liquid to keep the sauce moist if necessary.

When the pasta is cooked, drain and return it to the pan. Add the pepper sauce, salt and lots of black pepper. Stir thoroughly and serve.

Vegetarian Chilli - 390 kcal

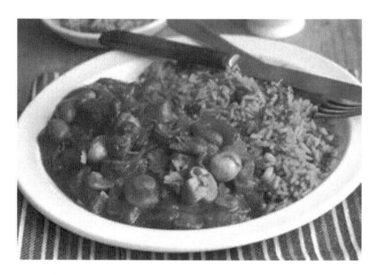

This is high in calories because of the rice. If you want to eat it without the rice then the calorie count drops to only 125 calories for the chilli. You could have it with a green salad or for a more substantial meal try putting it in a flatbread with some lettuce which will only total 225 calories.

390 calories per serving
Preparation - 5 minutes
Cooking - 20 minutes

Ingredients

- ½ red chilli
- 100g / 3½ oz mushrooms

- 1 garlic clove
- ½ tsp cumin
- 200g / 7 oz can chopped tomatoes
- 200g / 7 oz can red kidney beans

To serve

- 75g / 2½ oz cooked brown rice

Method

Fry the finely chopped garlic and red chilli in 1 tbsp of olive oil with the cumin. Add the chopped mushrooms and cook for about 4 minutes more but add some water if the mushrooms do not release enough liquid.

Add the chopped tomatoes and kidney beans, stir and cook for another 10 minutes on a very low heat making sure you stir often or it will stick. Serve with the cooked brown rice.

Sweet Potato Curry - 350 kcal

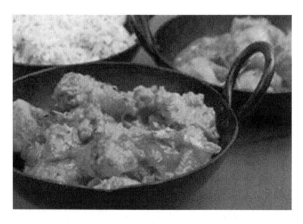

This is a very easy one-pot meal that you will cook again and again just because it is so delicious and quick to do. You will even consider having it on your non fasting days with rice and a naan.

350 calories per serving
Preparation - 10 minutes
Cooking - 30 minutes

Ingredients

- 50g / 2 oz red lentils
- 225ml / 8 fl oz / 1 cup vegetable stock
- 1 small onion
- 1 medium tomato
- ½ tsp turmeric
- ½ tsp garam masala
- 1 small red chilli

- 1 medium sweet potato
- 2 handfuls baby spinach

Method

Finely chop the onion and chilli and roughly chop the tomato. Peel and cube the sweet potato and shred the baby spinach.

Put the lentils, stock, onion, tomatoes, spices and the red chilli into a pan, bring to a simmer and cook for 10 minutes. Add the sweet potato and cook for a further 10 minutes or until done.

Stir in the shredded baby spinach and season to taste. When spinach is wilted, serve at once

218

Notes

FISH

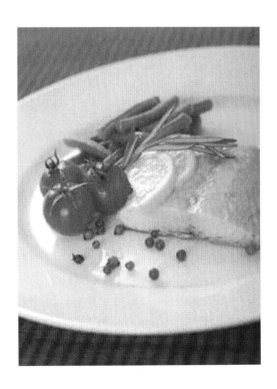

Fishcakes & Vege Stir Fry - 360 kcal

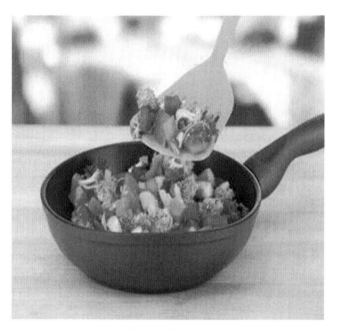

This is a very basic dish that started out being one of our staple meals for fasting days. I usually buy the melt in the middle luxury fishcakes and keep a couple of packs in the freezer. These are higher in calories than the standard bought fishcakes but they are much more satisfying. However any shop bought fishcake will do, just check the packaging for calories.

360 calories per serving
Preparation - 10 minutes
Cooking - 20 minutes

Ingredients

- 1 fishcake no more than 300 calories per fishcake.
- 1 medium courgette or zucchini
- 1 tomato
- 75g / 2½ oz broccoli florets
- 1 stick celery.
- 1 vegetable stock cube
- balsamic vinegar

Method

Cook fishcakes in oven as directed. In the meantime chop all the vegetables into bite size pieces and stir fry with a dash of water and a splash of balsamic vinegar.

Crumble the stock cube into the mix and cook until the vegetables are just tender or as liked. You shouldn't need additional seasoning because the stock cube is quite seasoned.

Fruity Fish Kebabs - 350 kcal

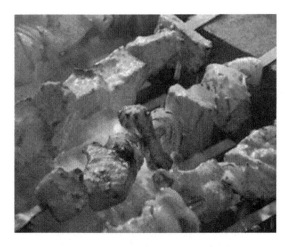

Any firm fish can be used to make these skewers but the combination of white and pink make the taste and look something special. You could also try it with tuna for a meatier taste.

350 calories per serving
Preparation - 15- 20 minutes
Cooking - 7-10 minutes

Ingredients

- 125g / 4½ oz firm fish such as Monkish or Cod
- 125g / 4½ oz thick salmon fillet
- 1 small orange
- ½ small grapefruit
- fresh bay leaves

For the marinade

- ½ tsp grated lemon rind
- 1 tbsp lemon juice
- ½ tsp runny honey
- 1 garlic clove

Method

Crush the garlic and mix with the lemon juice, rind and honey and set aside. Skin the fish and cut into 4 pieces each type making 8 pieces in all.

Using a knife, remove the peel and pith from the grapefruit and orange and carefully cut out each segment. Try to make sure you have cut out all pith and linking membranes.

Thread 2 skewers alternating the two fish types, bay leaves, grapefruit and orange segments. Place the skewers in a long shallow dish or plate and pour over the marinade you made earlier. Cover and chill for a couple of hours, turning them over in the marinade every so often.

To cook, preheat a grill to medium heat, place a piece of foil on the grill pan or barbecue and grill for about 8 minutes, turning half way through. Make sure the fish is fully cooked.

Serve with a fresh green salad and baby tomatoes.

Olive & Anchovy Pasta - 385 kcal

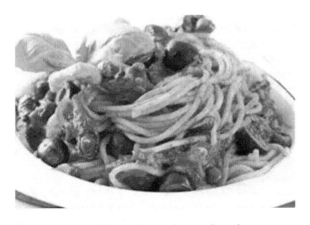

This is very quick and simple meal and you can use any pasta with the sauce. Tagliatelli or spaghetti will work best because the sauce will stick to it for a more enjoyable taste.

385 calories per serving
Preparation - 20 minutes
Cooking - 30 minutes

Ingredients

- 1 cal oil spray
- 1 small red onion
- 2 anchovy fillets
- Pinch chilli flakes
- 1 garlic clove
- 100g / 3½ oz canned chopped tomatoes
- 1 tbsp tomato puree
- 60g / 2¼ oz fresh tagliatelli or other pasta

- 10g / ¼ oz each of green and black pitted olives
- 1 tsp capers
- 1 sun-dried tomatoes
- salt and pepper

Method

Finely chop the onion and garlic. Roughly chop or slice the olives and sun-dried tomatoes. Drain the anchovies and drain and rinse the capers.

Heat 15 pumps of the oil spray in a pan and sauté the onion, anchovies and chilli flakes for 10 minutes until starting to turn brown, add the garlic and cook for a further 30 seconds. Add the canned tomatoes and puree and bring to a simmer and cook on a low heat for about 10 minutes.

In the meantime, cook the pasta as directed until al-dente or firm but not hard usually about 4 minutes depending on pasta type..

Add the olives, sun-dried tomatoes and capers to the sauce. Simmer for a further 3 minutes and then season to taste.

Drain the pasta, return to the pan and add the sauce, stirring until pasta and sauce are fully combined. Serve at once.

Tuna, Salmon & Couscous - 360 kcal

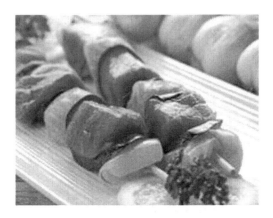

Tuna steak meat is ideal for threading on to sticks for kebabs and cooks really well on either the grill or barbecue.

360 calories per serving
Preparation – 5 minutes + 10 minutes marinating
Cooking - 5 minutes

Ingredients

- 1 piece tuna approx 60g / 2¼ oz
- 1 piece salmon approx 60g / 2¼ oz
- 1 small courgette or zucchini
- 1 tbsp harrissa paste
- 1 lemon
- 50g / 2 oz couscous
- 100ml / 3½ oz / scant ½ cup vegetable stock

- 1 tsp cumin
- small bunch mint, chopped

Method

Cut the tuna and salmon into fairly large chunks. Cut the lemon in half and squeeze the juice from one half and cut the other into wedges for serving later. Mix the harissa paste with 2 tsp lemon juice and coat the fish pieces with it. Leave to marinate for 10 minutes.

Bring the stock to the boil and add the cumin, stir and pour over the couscous. Cover and leave to stand for 5 minutes and then fluff up.

Slice the courgette/zucchini into medium thickness slices diagonally into long pieces.

Thread the fish and vegetable slices alternately and evenly between 4 skewers and grill or barbecue for 2 minutes each side or until the fish is cooked through.

Mix the remaining lemon juice and mint with the couscous and serve with the fish kebabs and the lemon wedges and a green salad.

Tuna Steak &Vege Mash - 325 kcal

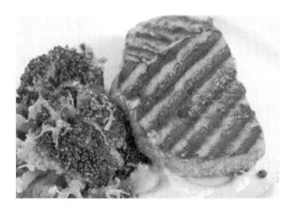

Sweet Potato is actually slightly higher in calories and carbs than white potatoes so you can have either. Personally I prefer the taste of the sweet potato and carrot mash but it's your choice. Using carrot to bulk up the mash saves you calories. If you do use white potatoes, make sure you only have the same combined weight. This mash also freezes well so you might consider making bigger batches for convenience.

325 calories per serving
***Mash is suitable for freezing
Preparation - 10 minutes
Cooking - 20 minutes

Ingredients

- 1 tuna steak approx 125g / 4½ oz each
- 1 sweet Potato - 200g / 7 oz peeled weight

- 1 medium carrot
- 1 medium tomato
- 100g / 4 oz of Broccoli florets
- 1 garlic clove

Method

Peel and chop sweet potato into largish chunks and the carrots into smaller slices as they take longer to cook. Boil in lightly salted water until soft, about 10-15 minutes depending on size, then mash with a little seasoning but no butter.

Oven bake the tuna sprayed with oil and water mixture for about 20 minutes or if you prefer, griddle for about 10 minutes turning over half way through cooking.

Cut the tomato in half and place in another dish. Peel and slice the garlic and poke the slivers into the flesh of the tomatoes. Drizzle with a tiny amount of olive oil and some freshly ground pepper and bake for about 15 minutes.

Steam or microwave the broccoli as liked and serve with the tuna, mash and baked tomatoes.

Tuna Steak & Vegetables - 385 kcal

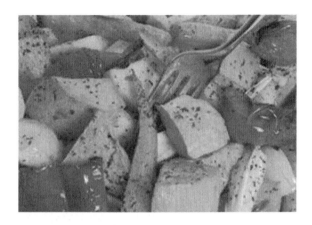

385 calories per serving
Preparation - 10 minutes
Cooking - 25 - 30 minutes

Ingredients

- 1 x 125g / 4½ oz tuna steak
- 1 small onion
- 1 small parsnip
- 1 medium carrot
- ½ small butternut squash
- 1 clove of garlic
- ½ x 400g / 14 oz tin of Chickpeas
- 1 tsp olive oil
- Juice of ½ lime
- 100ml / 3½ fl oz / scant ½ cup of water
- Small handful basil leaves

Method

Preheat the oven to 200°C/gas mark 6.

Peel and chop the onions, parsnips and carrots into bite sized pieces, not too big or they won't cook. Peel and slice the garlic and drain and rinse the chickpeas. Heat the oil in a large roasting dish in the pre-heated oven. While the oil is heating up, chop, de-seed and peel the squash, cutting it into 2-cm chunks.

Add the onions, parsnips, carrots and garlic to the roasting dish, stir to coat them in the oil and spread them out. Bake for 10 minutes. Then add the squash, together with the lime juice and mix well.

Roast for a further 15 minutes and then add the drained chickpeas and the water. Continue cooking for a further 10 minutes and then stir in the basil leaves.

During the final 10 minutes cooking time cook the tuna steak according to how you like it over a medium heat on a griddle or frying pan brushed very lightly with oil.

Put a portion of the roasted vegetables on each plate, topped by the tuna steak and serve with a green salad

Notes

MEAT & POULTRY

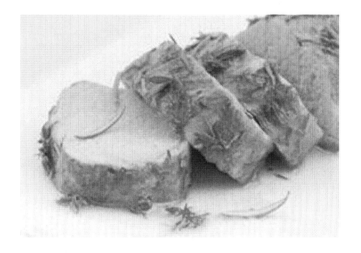

Beef & Courgette Bake - 330 kcal

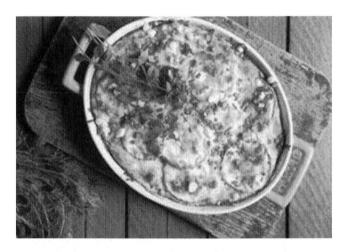

This dish uses courgette and tomatoes in place of high calorie potatoes for a type of cottage pie or lasagna. Freezes well so you can cook more and have it another day but will feed the whole family if you increase the ingredients. Serve with some steamed vegetables and for the non fasting family members add some new potatoes or some crusty bread.

330 calories per serving
***Suitable for freezing
Preparation – 10 minutes
Cooking – 60-70 minutes

Ingredients

- 90g/3 oz low fat minced or ground beef
- 1 small onion
- ½ tsp dried mixed herbs
- 1 tsp flour
- 75ml / 3 fl oz / ⅓ cup beef stock
- 1 tsp tomato paste
- 1 medium tomato
- 1 medium courgette / zucchini
- 2 tsp cornflour
- 75ml or 3 fl oz / ⅓ cup skimmed milk
- 50ml or 2 fl oz or ¼ cup low-fat fromage frais
- 1 egg yolk
- 1 tbsp grated parmesan cheese

Method

Pre-heat the oven to 190°C or 375°F or Gas 5

Finely chop the onion and thinly slice the tomatoes and courgettes.

Fry the beef and onion without any added oil for 5 minutes until browned all over. Drain off any surplus fat and then stir in the dried herbs, flour, stock and tomato paste and bring to a simmer. Cook for 30 minutes until the mixture is sauce like.

Transfer to a suitable oven-proof dish relative to the portion you have cooked. Cover with a layer of sliced tomatoes and then courgettes. Leave to one side.

Mix the cornflour with a little of the milk to form a paste. Heat the remaining milk in either a saucepan or the microwave until just coming up to boil. Add the cornflour paste and whip until it thickens and either stir over the heat for 1-2 minutes or pop back in the microwave for another minute. Remove from heat and beat in the fromage frais and the egg yolk.

Cover the layers of the meat dish with the white sauce, sprinkle with the grated parmesan cheese and bake in the oven for 20-25 minutes or until crisp and golden on top.

Notes

Chicken Lasagne - 390 kcal

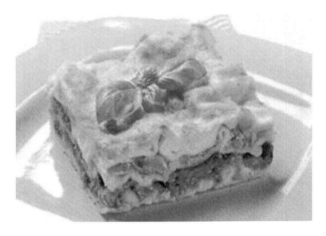

An easy dish to cook for a dinner or late supper and it is very filling.

390 calories per serving
***Suitable for freezing
Preparation - 15 minutes
Cooking - 50-60 minutes

Ingredients

- 90g/3oz frozen chopped spinach thawed
- 100g / 3½ oz cooked chicken breast
- 1 sheet fresh lasagna
- 1½ tsp cornflour
- 110ml/4 fl oz/1 cup skimmed milk
- 1 tbsp parmesan cheese grated
- 100g / 3½ oz canned chopped tomatoes

- 1 small onion
- 1 garlic clove
- 50 ml / 2 fl oz / ¼ cup white wine
- 1 tbsp tomato puree
- ½ tsp dried tarragon

Method

Chop the cooked chicken and finely chop the onion and garlic clove. Make the tomato sauce by heating the tomatoes, onion, garlic, wine, tomato paste and dried tarragon in a pan. Bring to a simmer and cook for 20 minutes until nice and thick. Season with salt and pepper and set aside.

Meanwhile, make sure the spinach is well drained and if necessary place on kitchen paper and mop until most of the water had gone.

Put half the spinach into a suitable sized baking dish, one that will take half a sheet of lasagna and season well. Cover the spinach with half the cooked chicken then half a sheet of lasagna, then half the tomato sauce. Repeat

Make a white sauce by mixing the cornflour with a little of the milk and then add the rest of the milk to the paste. Heat either in a small saucepan for 2-3 minutes or in the microwave until the sauce is thick but not solid.

Cover the top lasagna sheet with the white sauce, sprinkle the grated parmesan on top and bake for 25 minutes at 200C/400F/Gas 6 until the top is golden and bubbling. Serve with a green salad.

Although this recipe is really easy to do, I actually

double or quadruple the ingredients, make two or four meals and freeze the excess. Less work all round and I always have a standby in the freezer for lazy fasting days.

Notes

Chicken & Chips - 400 kcal

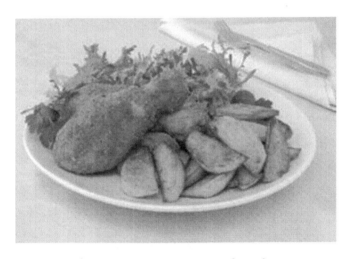

You can't usually have this type of meal on your fasting days but this is a low fat version that just about creeps into your allowance.

400 calories per serving
Preparation - 10 minutes
Cooking - 30-35 minutes

Ingredients

- 1 x 225g/8 oz baking potato
- ½ tbsp sunflower oil
- 1 tsp coarse sea salt
- 2 tsp plain flour
- ½ tsp paprika pepper
- 2 chicken drumsticks, no skin

- 1 small egg
- 1 tbsp water
- 1½ tbsp dry white breadcrumbs
- salt and pepper

Method

Pre-heat oven to 200°C / 400°F / Gas 6

Scrub the potato but do not peel and cut into 8 equal size wedges. Put into a bowl with the oil and toss well to coat all over. Put on a non stick baking sheet or tray, sprinkle with the sea salt.

In a bowl, mix the flour with the paprika and season well. Coat the chicken with the flour mixture and shake off any excess. Beat the egg with the water and pour onto a plate. On another plate spread out the breadcrumbs. Now dip the chicken into the egg and then the breadcrumbs, making sure you cover as much chicken as you can.

Place the chicken on another non stick tray and bake in the pre-heated oven, together with the potato wedges for 30-35 minutes, turning the chicken after 15 minutes.

When cooked and crispy, drain the potato wedges onto kitchen paper to remove excess oil and serve with the chicken and perhaps a spoonful of low fat relish of choice.

Chicken & Wild & Brown Rice
- 370 kcal

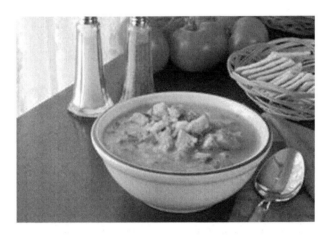

I love to cook a one pot dish because it is easier and saves on washing up. This dish is also very filling and nutritious because of the brown rice.

370 calories per serving
***Suitable for freezing
Preparation - 5 minutes
Cooking - 45-50 minutes

Ingredients

- 1 small onion
- 1 garlic clove
- 1 stick of celery
- 1 carrot
- 75ml / 3 fl oz / scant ½ cup chicken stock

- 90g / 3oz skinless chicken breasts
- 60g / 2 oz mixed brown and wild rice
- 100g / 3½ oz canned chopped tomatoes
- 1 medium courgette/zucchini
- salt and pepper

Method

Chop the onion, crush the garlic, slice the celery, dice the carrot and thinly slice the courgette.

Put the onion, garlic, celery and carrot in a large pan with the stock, bring to a simmer, cover and cook on a low heat for 5 minutes.

Slice the chicken into 2.5cm/ 1 inch cubes and add to the pan. Stir and cover again and cook for a further 5 minutes.

Add the rice and chopped tomatoes, season, bring back to the boil, cover and simmer gently for 20 minutes.

Stir in the sliced courgettes and carry on cooking for another 10 minutes but without the lid. Stir occasionally to prevent sticking, adding more water if it is getting too dry and the rice has not fully cooked. Serve with a green salad.

Deep South Turkey Steak - 355 kcal

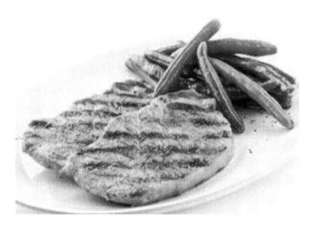

Turkey is one of the cheapest cuts of meat and really low in fat content so make the most of this with an easy to cook meal. Because you are having new potatoes, you won't realise this is a fasting day.

355 calories per serving
Preparation – 10 minutes
Cooking – 15-20 minutes

Ingredients

- 100g turkey steak fillet
- 150g / 6 oz small new potatoes
- 50g / 2oz runner beans
- 1 tbsp Cajun seasoning
- 1 cal oil spray
- Juice and zest of ½ lemon

- 1 garlic clove
- 1 medium tomato

Method

Trim and thickly slice the runner beans. De-seed and chop the tomato into chunks. Crush the garlic. Cook the new potatoes for 8 minutes, add the runner beans and cook for another 4 minutes.

While the potatoes and beans are cooking, press the Cajun seasoning onto both sides of the turkey streaks.

Heat 10 pumps of oil spray in a large non-stick frying pan and cook the turkey for 3-4 minutes each side until they start to go black. Sprinkle with the lemon juice and zest and cook to reduce. Remove from the pan and keep hot.

Drain the vegetables and heat another 10 pumps of oil in the pan. and stir in the potatoes, beans, garlic and tomatoes. Cook for about 2 minutes and serve with the turkey steak and any liquid from the pan.

Chicken & Orzo Pasta - 365 kcal

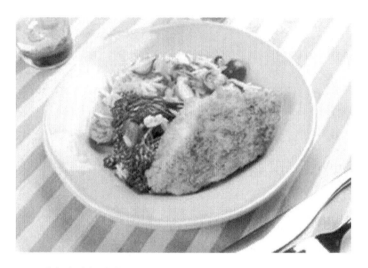

This is ideal for a barbecue or summer buffet because it can be eaten hot or cold. The pasta pushes up the calories a bit so try having just a salad if you are near your limit and deduct 150 calories.

365 calories per serving
Preparation - 10 minutes
Cooking - 20-25 minutes

Ingredients

- 1 x 125g/4oz boneless chicken breast
- 1 tsp clear honey
- 1 tsp soy sauce
- ½ tsp grated lemon rind
- 1 tsp lemon juice

- salt and pepper
- 45g / 1 ¾ oz Orzo pasta
- 3 cherry tomatoes
- 1 tsp olive oil
- 1 pinch chilli flakes

Method

Preheat the grill/broiler to medium

Skin the chicken and trim off any fat. Pat dry and score a criss-cross pattern on both sides of the breast but make sure you do not cut all the way through.

In a small bowl, mix the honey, soy sauce, lemon rind and juice and plenty of seasoning.

Put the chicken on the grill or barbecue rack and brush with half of the honey glaze. Cook for 10 minutes, turn the chicken over and brush with the rest of the glaze. Cook for another 10 minutes or until cooked through, depending on your barbecue heat.

While the chicken is grilling, cook the orzo according to the packet instructions, drain and mix in the olive oil and chilli flakes and season with black pepper and salt and keep warm.

Serve the pasta with the cooked chicken, halved cherry tomatoes some extra lemon zest and a green salad or steamed broccoli if liked.

Lamb Kebabs - 325 kcal

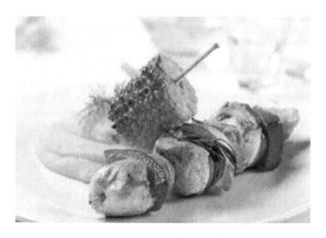

325 calories per serving
Preparation 10 minutes
Cooking - 15-25 minutes

Ingredients

- 200g / 7 oz lean lamb steaks
- ½ red pepper
- ½ green pepper
- 25g / 1 oz low-fat yoghurt
- 1 tsp olive oil
- 1 small onion
- several fresh sprigs of rosemary

Method

Cut the lamb into 2-cm cubes, removing any excess fat. Put the cubes into a bowl; pour over the yogurt and olive oil. Toss in the mixture making sure the lamb is fully covered. Cover and chill for at least 4 hours or overnight if you have time.

When ready, remove lamb from fridge, peel and cut the onion into quarters, chop the peppers into cubes and thread onto the skewers alternating lamb, peppers and onion. Metal skewers are fine but if using bamboo you should soak them first to avoid burning and the food sticking.

Cook them on a hot barbecue or under a pre-heated grill, laying them on a piece of foil and a few fresh sprigs of rosemary, until they are done to your taste.

Serve with a green salad and low calorie tzatsiki as a dressing.

Sausages in Batter - 325 kcal

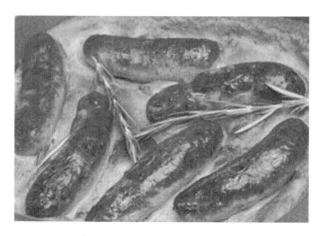

This is a low fat version of Toad in the Hole. You could use the Quorn or similar sausages if preferred but compare the calorie count.

325 calories per serving
Preparation 10 minutes
Cooking – 55-60 minutes

Ingredients

- ½ red onion
- 2 low fat pork sausages or quorn equivalent
- ½ tsp olive oil
- 25g / 1oz plain flour
- 1 medium egg
- 75ml / 3 fl oz / scant ½ cup skimmed milk
- ½ tsp creamed horseradish

- 150g / 5 oz broccoli
- 50g / 2 oz carrots

Method

Pre-heat the oven to 200°C / Gas 6

Cut the onion into wedges and separate the layers. Place in a small shallow non-stick tin or ceramic dish. Arrange the sausages on top of the onions, add the oil and roast for 20 minutes.

Meanwhile make the batter by beating the egg into the sifted flour and then add the milk a little at a time until all the lumps have gone and the batter is nice and smooth. Stir in the horseradish and season to taste. When the sausages have been cooking for the 20 minutes, drain any excess fat but leave a little in the pan. Pour the batter into the pan and put back in the oven for another 30 minutes or until golden and fluffy. Serve with the steamed broccoli and carrots.

Marinated Balsamic Beef - 350 kcal

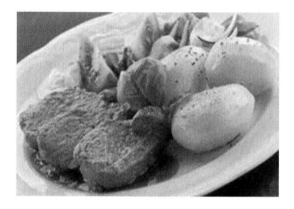

Use rump steak for this dish as it is fairly inexpensive especially if you can get it on offer. You could use cheaper cuts but I don't like chewy meat so would rather pay a little extra.

350 calories per serving
Preparation – 25 minutes (including marinating)
Cooking – 15-20 minutes

Ingredients

- 150g/7oz piece of rump streak
- 2 shallots
- 1 tbsp balsamic vinegar
- 125g/5oz new potatoes
- 125g / 4½ oz fresh washed spinach

Method

Place the beef in a shallow tray or dish. Finely chop the shallots and mix with the balsamic vinegar. Rub this all over the meat and marinate for 20 minutes.

Wash the potatoes and thickly slice. Cook in salted boiling water for 12-15 minutes or until just tender and remove from the heat.

Pop the spinach into the pan for a couple of minutes to wilt and then drain well and keep warm.

While the potatoes are cooking, grill or barbecue the marinated beef for 3-4 minutes each side depending on the thickness of the meat and your preference. Cook for longer if liked. Remove and wrap in foil for 5 minutes.

Slice the beef thinly across the grain and served on a bed of the potatoes and spinach. Sprinkle with a little balsamic vinegar and olive oil.

Pork & Plum Hotpot - 360 kcal

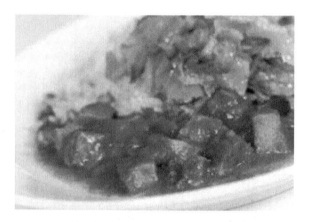

This is delicious especially when the plums are in season and are so sweet and inexpensive. The pasta makes it a little more substantial.

360 calories per serving
Preparation 10 minutes
Cooking – 35 – 40 minutes

Ingredients

- 100g / 3½ pork fillet
- 1 cal oil spray
- 1 garlic clove
- 50g / 1½ oz shallots
- 60g / 2oz plums
- 110ml / 4 fl oz / scant ½ cup chicken stock
- 15g / ½ oz of orzo pasta

Method

Halve the shallots, crush the garlic, halve and stone the plums, if large halve again.

Cut the pork into 2.5cm/1 inch pieces and in a large frying pan, fry the meat and the garlic and shallots in a few pumps of oil spray until browned all over.

Stir in the plums and stock, bring to the boil and simmer for about 10 minutes then add the pasta and cook for a further 10 minutes until the meat is cooked through and the pasta is soft. Add more stock if goes too dry before pasta is cooked.

Serve with a green salad or steamed broccoli or some crusty bread on a non fasting day.

Pork Stroganoff & Rice - 350 kcal

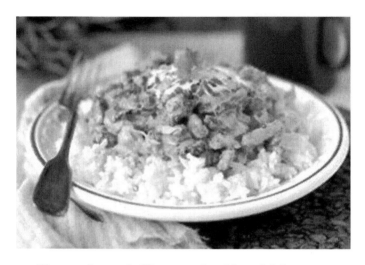

Use tender pork fillet to make this quick but delicious dish. The mushrooms and green pepper blend well with the tomato and yogurt sauce. If you eat it without the rice the calorie count drops to 195

350 calories per serving
Preparation - 10 minutes
Cooking - 30 minutes

Ingredients

- 90g / 3 oz lean pork fillet
- 1 cal oil spray
- ½ small onion
- 1 garlic clove – crushed
- 15g / ½ oz plain flour

- 2 tsp tomato puree
- 125 ml / 4 fl oz / ½ cup of chicken stock
- 40g / 1½ oz button mushrooms
- ½ medium green bell pepper
- ½ tsp ground nutmeg
- 1 tbsp low-fat natural yogurt
- salt & pepper

To serve

- 40g / 1½ oz basmati rice
- tbsp natural yogurt

Method

Chop the onion, slice the mushrooms and deseed and dice the green pepper. Trim the meat of all fat and skin and cut into 1cm or ½ inch slices.

Heat a large pan, add 10 pumps of the oil spray and fry the pork, garlic and onion for 5 minutes until meat is slightly browned. Add the flour and tomato paste and stir through, then add the stock, a little at a time and mix well.

Add the mushrooms, pepper, seasoning and nutmeg, bring back to the boil and simmer on a low heat for about 20 minutes.

Meanwhile cook the rice in a pan of boiling water for about 12 minutes or as directed on the packet. Drain and keep warm. Remove the Stroganoff from the heat, stir in the yogurt and serve with the rice in warmed bowls.

Steak & Mushroom Pie - 390 kcal

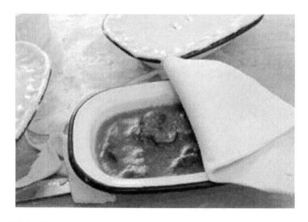

This is worth taking the time to prepare and cook because it is really uplifting when you are on a diet day.

390 calories per serving
Preparation - 25 minutes
Cooking - 50-55 minutes

Ingredients

- 1 small onion
- 1 small carrot
- 1 celery stick
- 1 tsp dried rosemary
- 100 ml / 3½ fl oz chicken stock
- 100g / 3½ oz small button mushrooms
- 75g / 3oz lean sirloin steak
- 1 tsp flour
- 50g / 2oz ready to roll puff pastry

- milk to glaze

Method

Finely chop the onion, carrot and celery. Trim any fat from the meat and cube into bite sized pieces.

Fry the onion, carrot and celery in a lidded saucepan for 5 minutes or until soft. Add a little stock to prevent sticking. Add the mushrooms, season and stir fry for a further 2 minutes and then using a slotted spoon, remove from pan.

Season the steak and fry the meat in a spray of oil until browned all over. Sprinkle with the flour, put the vegetables back in the pan and mix together. Pour over the stock and bring to the boil, reduce heat and simmer very gently for 30 minutes on a low heat.

As meat is cooking, roll out pastry to fit your single serving pie dish and preheat the oven to 180C / 160C fan / Gas Mark 4.

Fill the dish with the meat filling and cover with the pastry top press firmly down on the dish edges to seal. Cut a slit in top and brush lightly with the milk. Bake for 20-25 minutes until golden.

Serve with a good portion of steamed broccoli.

Tomato, Chicken & Orzo - 360 kcal

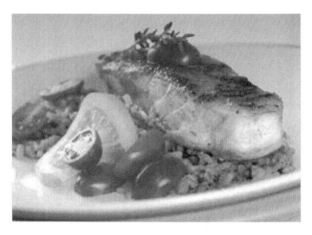

This is a simple and economical pasta dish that will leave you full as well as happy. Cook enough of the sauce to freeze for another fasting day; just don't cook the pasta until needed.

360 calories per serving
Preparation – 5 minutes
Cooking – 30 minutes

Ingredients

- 1 cal oil spray
- 1 boneless and skinless chicken breast
- ½ small onion
- 1 clove garlic
- 60 ml / 2 fl oz / ¼ cup chicken stock
- pinch chilli flakes

- 100g / 3½ oz canned chopped tomatoes
- 50g / 1oz dry weight orzo pasta

Method

Halve and finely slice the onion and garlic. Slice the chicken into long strips.

In a large pan heat 10 pumps of the oil spray and sauté the chicken until browned all over and remove from pan. Add the onion, garlic and chilli flakes and cook for about 5 minutes giving a couple more sprays of the oil if it looks too dry.

Add the tomatoes and stock to the pan and return the chicken. Season well and simmer for a further 10 minutes. While the sauce is simmering, cook the orzo pasta according to the pack and serve with the chicken

Notes

Snacks & Treats

Cheddars Cheese biscuits -- 20 kcal per biscuit
Crackers -- 32 kcal per biscuit
Rice Cakes -- 30 kcal per cake
Ryvita Crackers -- 27 kcal per cracker
Warburtons Thin -- 100 kcal per roll
1 small apple, flesh only -- 90 kcal

Fruit -- per 100g
apple -- 47
apricots -- 32
blackberries -- 25
cherries -- 48
clementines -- 40
cranberries -- 55
grapes -- 60
kiwi -- 49
melon - cantaloupe -- 19
melon - galia -- 24
melon - honeydew -- 28
melon - watermelon -- 31
nectarines - flesh only -- 40
oranges - flesh only -- 37

peaches -- 33
pears -- 40
pineapple -- 41
plums -- 36
raspberries -- 25
rhubarb -- 7
satsuma flesh only -- 36
strawberries -- 27
tangarine -- 35

Vegetables --
carrot sticks raw -- 35
cauliflower raw -- 34
celery raw -- 7
courgettes raw -- 18
cucumber -- 10
lettuce -- 16
mushrooms raw -- 13

Peppers, stalk & seeds removed
green - raw -- 15
red - raw -- 32
yellow - raw -- 26

Potatoes
potato - baked, flesh only -- 77
potatoes new boiled -- 70

Other Salad
radish -- 12

spinach -- 25
spring onions -- 23
mini corncobs -- 24
tomatoes -- 19
tomatoes - cherry -- 18

Calorie Counter

All calories given are for 100g or 100ml liquids

BEANS & LENTILS

Baked beans -- 83
Black Eye beans -- 455
Butter beans -- 270
Chickpeas -- 320
Flageolet beans -- 279
Haricot -- 69
Lentils (brown) -- 297
Lentils (green) -- 316
Lentils (red) -- 327
Lentils (yellow) -- 334
Lima butter beans -- 282
Pinto beans -- 309
Puy -- 307
Red kidney beans -- 311
Soybeans -- 375
White beans -- 285

BREADS
Baguette -- 242

Chapatti -- 278

Ciabatta -- 269

Gluten-free -- 282

Pita, white -- 265

Pumpernickel -- 183

Rye -- 242

Soda, brown -- 223

Sourdough -- 256

Spelt -- 241

Whole grain -- 260

Whole wheat -- 234

Bagels -- 256

Plain croissant -- 414

Crumpets -- 180

BREAKFAST CEREALS
All bran -- 334

Alpen -- 361

Dorset cereal muesli -- 356

Granola -- 432

Kallo milk choc rice cakes -- 495

Muesli (unsweetened) -- 353

Oatmeal -- 363

Porridge Oats -- 355

Porridge (ready to eat) per serving -- 95

Quaker Oat So Simple instant porridge -- 380

Special K -- 379

CAKES

Apple pie -- 262

Apple tart -- 265

Baklava -- 498

Brownies -- 419

Carrot cake, iced -- 359

Chewing gum, sugar-free -- 159

Chocolate (dark) -- 547

Chocolate (milk) -- 549

Chocolate (white) -- 567

Chocolate cake, iced -- 414

Chocolate chip cookies -- 499

Chocolate croissant -- 433

Chocolate mousse -- 174

Chocolate-covered raisins -- 418

Cinnamon buns -- 280

Crystallized ginger -- 351

Digestives Mcvities -- 478

Flapjacks, all-butter -- 457

Ice cream, vanilla -- 190

Lemon cake -- 366

Liquorice -- 325

Marshmallow -- 338

Meringue -- 394

Mince pies -- 398

Oatmeal raisin cookies -- 445

Pain aux raisins -- 335

Peppermints -- 395

Scones -- 366

Sherbet, lemon -- 390

Shortbread, all-butter -- 523

Sorbet, lemon -- 118

Tiramisu -- 263

Toffee -- 459

Yoghurt-covered dried fruit -- 447

CHEESE

Babybel -- 362

Babybel light -- 210

Boursin -- 405

Boursin light -- 140

Brie -- 320

Camembert -- 290

Cheddar cheese (low-fat) -- 263

Cheddar, mature, medium -- 410

Cottage cheese (low-fat) -- 72

Cottage cheese, plain -- 101

Cream cheese (low-fat) -- 109

Danish blue -- 342

Dolcelatte -- 395

Edam -- 341

Emmenthal -- 370

Feta -- 250

Goat cheese, soft -- 324

Gouda -- 377

gruyere -- 396

Parmesan cheese (fresh, grated) -- 389

Parmesan cheese (previously grated) -- 389

Philadelphia cream cheese (low-fat) -- 111

Philadelphia cream cheese (normal) -- 245

Ricotta -- 134
Roquefort -- 368

DRIED FRUIT
Açai (dried berry powder) 1G -- 5
Cherries (glacé) -- 313
Dried apple -- 310
Dried apricot -- 196
Dried banana chips -- 523
Dried blueberries -- 313
Dried cranberries -- 346
Dried dates (pitted) -- 303
Dried figs -- 229
Dried mango -- 268
Dried prunes -- 151
Raisins -- 292

DRINKS
Apple juice -- 44
Beer, bitter -- 32
Beer, lager -- 43
Cappuccino, whole milk -- 37
Cappuccino, skimmed milk -- 22
Champagne -- 76
Coca cola -- 43
Coffee (black) -- 0
Coffee (with semi-sk milk) -- 7
Coke (diet) -- 0
Coke (normal) -- 43
Cordial (elderflower) -- 27

Cordial (lime) -- 24

Espresso -- 20

Gin and tonic -- 70

Ginger ale (dry) -- 34

Hot chocolate -- 59

Hot chocolate (low-cal) -- 19

Hot milk and honey (semi-sk) -- 58

Innocent smoothie (mango) -- 56

Innocent smoothie (strawberry/banana) -- 53

Latte (skimmed milk) -- 29

Latte (whole milk) -- 54

Lemonade -- 47

Lime juice -- 23

Macchiato (skimmed milk) -- 26

Macchiato (whole milk) -- 30

Milkshakes (strawberry) -- 67

Orange juice -- 42

Orange squash -- 10

Pear juice -- 43

Red wine -- 68

Ribena -- 43

Sparkling water -- 0

Sprite -- 44

Tea (black) -- 0

Tea (chai latte, semi-sk) -- 70

Tea (green) (herbal) -- 0

Vodka tonic -- 71

Wheatgrass (frozen juice) -- 17

White wine -- 66

EGGS

Egg whites -- 50

Eggs (fried) -- 187

Eggs (omelette) -- 173

Eggs (poached) -- 145

Eggs (scrambled) -- 155

Eggs (boiled) -- 147

FISH & SEAFOOD

Anchovies, canned in oil, drained -- 191

Calamari (battered, frozen) -- 200

Cod steaks, grilled -- 95

Crab, boiled -- 128

Dover sole -- 78

Eels, jellied -- 98

Fish, unbreaded -- 76

Haddock (fillets) -- 74

Halibut -- 100

Herring, raw or grilled -- 190

Kipper fillets, smoked -- 198

Kippers, grilled -- 255

Lemon sole, steamed -- 91

Mackerel (fillets) -- 204

Mussels -- 92

Plaice, steamed -- 93

Prawns, boiled -- 99

Prawns, king, cooked & peeled -- 76

Salmon (canned) -- 131

Salmon, fillet, grilled -- 169

Sardines (fresh) -- 165

Sardines (tinned, in water) -- 179

Scallops -- 83

Sea bass (fillets) -- 133

Seafood (unbreaded) -- 76

Sushi -- 156

Tuna (canned) -- 108

Tuna (fresh) -- 137

FRUIT

Apples -- 51

Apricots -- 32

Bananas -- 103

Blackberries -- 26

Blueberries -- 60

Cherries -- 52

Clementines -- 41

Compote (apple & blackberry) -- 107

Cranberries -- 42

Figs -- 230

Goji berries -- 313

Grapefruit -- 30

Grapes -- 66

Kiwi -- 55

Lemon -- 20

Limes -- 12

Mandarin -- 35

Melon -- 29

Nectarines -- 44

Oranges -- 40

Papaya -- 40

Peaches -- 37
Pears -- 41
Pineapple -- 43
Plums -- 39
Pomegranate -- 55
Prunes (tinned) -- 90
Raspberries -- 30
Satsuma's -- 31
Smoothies (strawberry/banana) -- 51
Strawberries -- 28
Tangerines -- 39
Watermelon -- 33

GRAINS
Barley -- 364
Buckwheat -- 343
Buckwheat noodles -- 363
Bulgar -- 334
Corn (popping) -- 339
Cous cous -- 358
Cream crackers -- 437
Matzo crackers -- 381
Millet -- 354
Noodles (instant) -- 450
Oats -- 369
Oat cakes -- 440
Ryvita (original) -- 350
Quinoa -- 375
Ramen noodles -- 361

RICE
Arborio rice -- 354
Basmati -- 350
Brown rice -- 340
Jasmine -- 352
Long grain -- 355
Paella -- 349
Short grain -- 351
Uncle Ben's white rice (long grain) -- 344
Wild rice -- 353

Rice cakes -- 379
Rice noodles -- 373
Rye -- 331
Spelt -- 314
Tortilla -- 307
Vermicelli noodles -- 354
Wheat berries -- 326
Whole grain cereal -- 345
Whole grain pasta -- 326
Whole wheat cereal -- 359
Whole wheat pasta -- 326

HERBS & SPICES – all 1g
Basil -- 0
Cinnamon -- 3
Cloves -- 3
Coriander -- 0
Cumin -- 4
Ginger -- 1

Lemongrass -- 1
Mint -- 0
Nutmeg -- 4
Oregano -- 3
Paprika -- 3
Parsley -- 0
Pepper -- 3
Rosemary -- 0
Saffron -- 3
Sage -- 3
Tamarind paste -- 1.5
Tarragon -- 0
Thyme -- 2
Turmeric -- 3

MEAT

Bacon -- 244
Beef, lean -- 116
Burger (lamb) -- 267
Burger (beef) -- 283
Chicken breast, skinless -- 105
Chicken thigh, skinless -- 163
Chipolata sausage -- 267
Chorizo sausage -- 348
Duck breast, skinless -- 92
Goose -- 356
Guinea fowl -- 158
Ham, lean -- 104
Ham (pre-packaged, sliced) -- 118
Lamb chops -- 260

Lamb loin -- 231

Lamb sausages -- 260

Liver (chicken) -- 122

Minced beef -- 184

Minced lamb -- 235

Minced pork -- 140

Pâté -- 322

Pork, lean -- 117

Pork sausage -- 272

Rabbit -- 137

Salami -- 352

Shrimp -- 65

Stewing beef -- 121

Stewing lamb -- 175

Turkey, skinless -- 103

Wild game, skinless (venison) -- 101

MILK & CREAM
per 100g or 100ml liquid

Almond milk -- 24

Goats milk (whole) -- 61

Greek yoghurt -- 132

Milk (whole) -- 64

Milk (semi skimmed) -- 50

Milk (1%) -- 41

Milk (skim) -- 35

Rice milk -- 46

Soy milk -- 42

Clotted cream -- 586
Crème fraiche (low-fat) -- 79
Crème fraiche (normal) -- 299
Custard -- 118
Double Cream -- 496
Fromage frais -- 105
Fruit yoghurt -- 94
Single Cream -- 193
Sour cream (low-fat) -- 104
Sour cream (normal) -- 192
Whipped cream -- 368
Yoghurt (low-fat, with active cultures) -- 66

NUTS
Almond (ground) -- 618
Almonds (flaked) -- 641
Almonds (whole) -- 613
Brazils -- 680
Cashews -- 583
Hazelnuts -- 660
Macadamias -- 748
Nuts (mixed, unsalted) -- 661
Peanuts -- 561
Pecans -- 698
Pine nuts -- 688
Pistachio -- 584
Walnuts -- 703

OILS & FATS
per 100g or 100ml liquid

Butter (unsalted) -- 739
Butter (salted) -- 739
Corn oil -- 829
Flaxseed oil -- 813
Flora -- 410
Hemp oil -- 837
Lard -- 899
Margarine -- 735
Olive oil -- 823
Olive oil spread -- 543
Rapeseed oil -- 825
Sunflower oil -- 828
Vegetable oil -- 827

PICKLES

Black olives (pitted, drained) -- 154
Capers -- 32
Chutney, tomato -- 141
Cornichons -- 34
Gherkins -- 38
Jalapeño -- 18
Piccalilli sauce -- 80
Pickled onions -- 36

SANDWICHES

Cheese and chutney -- 228
Egg and cress -- 232
Ham and cheese -- 288
Tuna salad -- 221

SAUCES/DIPS/DRESSINGS
per 100g or 100ml liquid

Savoury
Barbecue sauce -- 144

Béarnaise sauce -- 580

Bolognaise sauce (no meat) -- 50

Gravy (beef, readymade) -- 45

Heinz salad cream -- 333

Hollandaise sauce -- 239

HP brown sauce -- 119

Lea & Perrins -- 115

Marmite -- 252

Mayonnaise (low-fat) -- 93

Mustard (Dijon) -- 160

Mustard (English) -- 167

Mustard (grain) -- 159

Pesto -- 431

Roasted aubergine spread/dip -- 102

Roasted red pepper spread/dip -- 235

Salad dressing (balsamic) -- 209

Salad dressing (Caesar no fat) -- 61

Salad dressing (olive oil and lemon) -- 439

Salad dressing (low-calorie) -- 68

Soy sauce -- 105

Sundried tomatoes -- 167

Taramasalata -- 516

Tartare sauce -- 358

Tikka masala sauce -- 133

Tomato and basil sauce -- 60

Tomato ketchup -- 102

Tzatzkiki -- 137

Vegemite -- 189

Vinegar (balsamic) -- 138

Vinegar (red wine) -- 23

Vinegar (white wine) -- 22

Sweet

Caramel sauce -- 389

Chocolate sauce -- 367

Cranberry sauce -- 192

Honey -- 334

Icing -- 405

Jam (strawberry) -- 258

Maple syrup -- 265

Marmalade -- 266

Nutella -- 529

Treacle 100G 294 -- 294

SAVOURY SNACKS

Breadsticks -- 408

Cheese straws -- 520

French fries (oven-baked) -- 260

Meat pies -- 293

Muffins (blueberry) -- 387

Pizza (Margherita) -- 258

Popcorn (salty) -- 520

Popcorn (sweet) -- 493

Potato chips (ready salted) -- 529

Quiche Lorraine -- 261

Peanuts (unsalted) -- 561
Salted peanuts -- 621
Salted mixed nuts -- 667
Samosas (vegetable) -- 225
Sausage roll -- 340
Vegetable chips -- 502

SEEDS
Chia seeds -- 422
Hemp seeds -- 437
Pumpkin seeds -- 590
Sesame seeds -- 616
Sunflower seeds -- 591
Flaxseed -- 495

SOUPS – per 100ml liquid
Bouillon -- 7
Carrot and coriander -- 35
Chicken noodle -- 35
Chowder -- 53
Cream of mushroom (Heinz) -- 50
Leek and potato -- 53
Light broth -- 36
Lobster bisque -- 68
Miso -- 22
Onion -- 45
Passata -- 31
Tomato (Heinz) -- 59
Tomato and basil -- 40
Vegetable -- 45

SWEETS

Cadbury's dairy milk -- 525

Green and Black's 70% chocolate -- 575

Green and Black's 85% chocolate -- 630

Haribo -- 344

Hob Nobs – Mcvities -- 473

Jaffa cakes -- 377

Lindt 70% chocolate -- 540

Tic Tacs -- 391

Wine gums -- 325

VEGETABLES

Artichoke (globe) -- 24

Artichoke (Jerusalem) -- 73

Asparagus -- 27

Aubergine sliced and griddled/grilled -- 18

Avocado -- 193

Beans - green

Trimmed raw -- 24

Trimmed , boiled -- 22

Canned -- 24

Frozen, whole -- 25

Frozen, sliced -- 27

Runner beans, trimmed, boiled -- 18

Bean sprouts -- 32

Beetroot -- 38

Bok Choy -- 15

Broad beans
Canned -- 82

Frozen, boiled -- 81

Fresh, shelled -- 77

Broccoli -- 32

Brussel sprouts -- 43

Cabbage -- 29

Carrot -- 34

Cauliflower -- 35

Celeriac -- 17

Celery -- 8

Chard -- 17

Chicory -- 19

Corn - see Sweetcorn

Courgette -- 18

Cucumber -- 10

Endive -- 17

Fennel -- 14

Garlic -- 106

Kale -- 33

Leeks -- 23

Lettuce -- 15
Hearts of Romaine -- 16

Iceberg -- 14

Mediterranean mixed -- 19

Mixed leaf -- 17

Rocket -- 24

Round -- 15

Mushrooms
Closed cup -- 16
Oyster -- 8
Portobello -- 13
Shiitake -- 27
Shiitake Dried -- 296

Onion (red) -- 38
Onion (white) -- 38
Peas, garden (frozen) -- 86
Peas, petit pois -- 52

Peppers
Chilli, green -- 20
Green, stalk & seeds removed -- 15
Jalapenos, green, sliced -- 24
Jalapenos, red, sliced -- 69
Mixed peppers, sliced, frozen -- 28
Red, stalk & seeds removed -- 32
Yellow, stalk & seeds removed -- 26

Potato (white) -- 79
Radicchio -- 19
Radish -- 13
Radish White (Mooli) -- 15
Ratatouille canned -- 50
Spinach -- 25
Spinach frozen, boiled -- 21
Squash -- 40

Sweetcorn
Giant baby cobs green giant -- 28
Mini corncobs canned -- 23
Mini corncobs fresh/frozen boiled -- 24
On the cob -- 110

Sweetcorn kernals
Canned, drained, re-heated -- 122
Frozen -- 93
Niblets with peppers (Green Giant) -- 82
Niblets, canned (Green Giant) -- 100
Niblets, naturally sweet (Green Giant) -- 77
Niblets, salad crisp (Green Giant) -- 70

Sweet potatoes -- 93
Swiss chard -- 19
Tomato -- 20
Turnip -- 24
Watercress -- 26

VEGETARIAN
Tofu -- 70
Quorn (chicken-style pieces) -- 114
Cauldron sausages -- 163

About the Author

Best Selling author Liz Armond was born and educated in London, UK. She has been an active student of fitness and nutrition for over 30 years. She has always tried to lead a healthy lifestyle and looks for ways to get healthier and live longer. After trying out the 5.2 diet and having great success she put together her favorite recipes adapted for the 5:2 and published her complete series of cookbooks suitable for every diet.

Liz is now an enthusiastic advocate for this proven diet and is a firm believer that following this diet and maintaining a healthy lifestyle will achieve her goal of living a long and happy life.

She is married with two children and is an enthusiastic golfer, rambler and is keen but not yet proficient in yoga and mediation. She also loves to ski whenever possible.

Other Books by Author

Recipes for the 5:2 Fast Diet
The Fast Diet Cookbook
Vegetarian Recipes for the 5:2 Fast Diet
Vegetarian & Gluten Free for the 5:2 Fast
Diet
Gluten Free for the 5:2 Fast Diet
5:2 Diet Breakfast Recipes
5:2 Diet Meal Plans & Recipes
5:2 Diet Meals for One Cookbook
Vegetarian Meals for One for the Fast Diet

Fasting Your Way to Health
Meditation for Beginners

Disclaimer and/or Legal Notices:

Every effort has been made to accurately represent this book and it's potential. Results vary with every individual, and your results may or may not be different from those depicted. No promises, guarantees or warranties, whether stated or implied, have been made that you will produce any specific result from this book. Your efforts are individual and unique, and may vary from those shown. Your success depends on your efforts, background and motivation.

The material in this publication is provided for educational and informational purposes only and is not intended as medical advice. The information contained in this book should not be used to diagnose or treat any illness, metabolic disorder, disease or health problem. Always consult your physician or health care provider before beginning any nutrition or exercise program. Use of the programs, advice, and information contained in this book is at the sole choice and risk of the reade

52259467R00168

Made in the USA
San Bernardino, CA
15 August 2017